*ten*minute
toning
FOR
bums
&tums

Sally Jones & Ellen Dupont

This is a Parragon Book
This edition published in 2005

Parragon
Queen Street House
4 Queen Street
Bath BA1 1 HE, UK

Produced by the Bridgewater Book Company Ltd

Photographer: Mike Hemsley at Walter Gardiner

ISBN: 1-40546-358-9

Printed in Indonesia

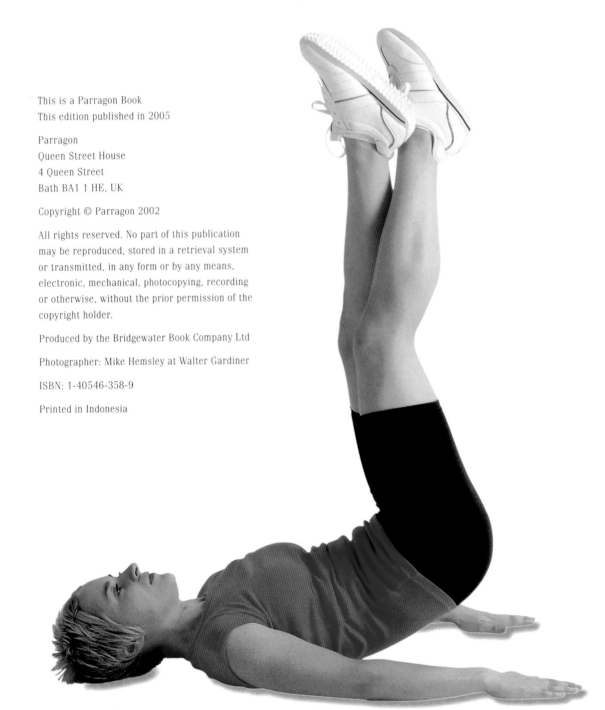

Contents

Introduction

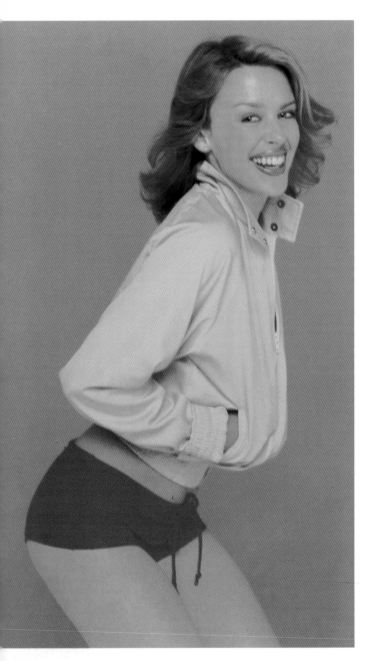

JUST DO IT! It's a short, simple slogan, but if you frequently ask the question 'Does my bum look big in this?', or you only dream of having a flat tummy, then it's time you did something about it. And when you know it can take just ten minutes to tone up and trim down, there's really no excuse not to get going.

Bums are big news. Images of beautiful behinds – whether it's the 'pert' bottom of singer Kylie Minogue or the curvaceous one of singer/actress Jennifer Lopez – are often splashed across the pages of our daily newspapers. There's no denying that a lean, toned, shapely bottom is sexier and more appealing than one that's not. Most women don't want a bottom that sags. They want it to be fit, firm and fabulous – and so do men!

As for our tums, this is the one part of the body that we like the least. Few women have a naturally flat stomach. The lower region of our body is where we tend to store extra fat, and pregnancy can take a toll on our waistlines, leaving us with a bulging tummy. Only by working the abdominal muscles correctly and regularly will 'the battle of the bulge' be won and a flatter, firmer midriff achieved.

The toning exercises in this ten-minute programme target the bum and tum areas.

To keep you inspired and motivated, visualise yourself with a pert bottom and flat tummy like Kylie Minogue's.

Take the time to learn how to do them correctly, perfect your technique, then practice them on a regular basis. Once you're familiar with the movements, you can create a programme that fits into your own lifestyle, designed to concentrate on the areas that you feel need the most work. As you begin to see an improvement, you'll be motivated to continue. For the very best results, combine this muscular strength programme with some form of regular cardiovascular exercise, and follow a sensible eating plan.

When it comes to losing weight, fad diets don't work. You might have success on a diet for the period of time that you're on it, but more often than not, when you've completed the programme, the weight comes back on. The only solution is to follow a sensible, healthy eating plan that can be maintained for a lifetime. Begin by making a few small but significant changes – reduce your intake of sugar, salt and fat, eat more fibre, and include at least five servings of fresh fruit and vegetables a day. 'Everything in moderation' is a good slogan to live by. Try to develop and appreciate a balanced and consistent approach to eating – and exercise.

The goals of this programme are simple: to change your eating habits for life and to start exercising regularly for a shapelier bum and flatter tum. One thing to remember about your body is that the way you look is largely down to genetics – but although big bums and thick thighs may run in the family, you can still work on creating the best version of your own body. It's never too late to start, so don't sit there thinking about it any more – JUST DO IT!

However busy your life is, it will take only a little time to create the exercise programme that is ideal for you.

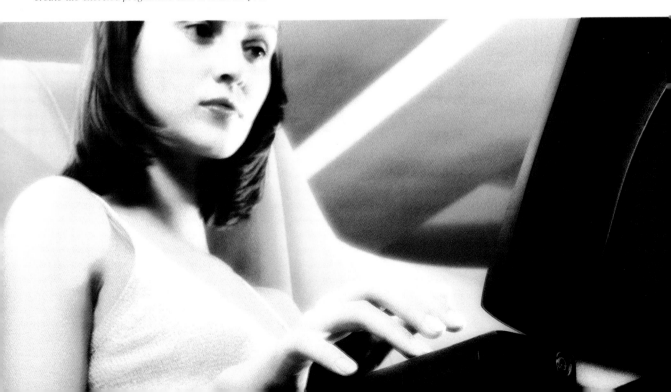

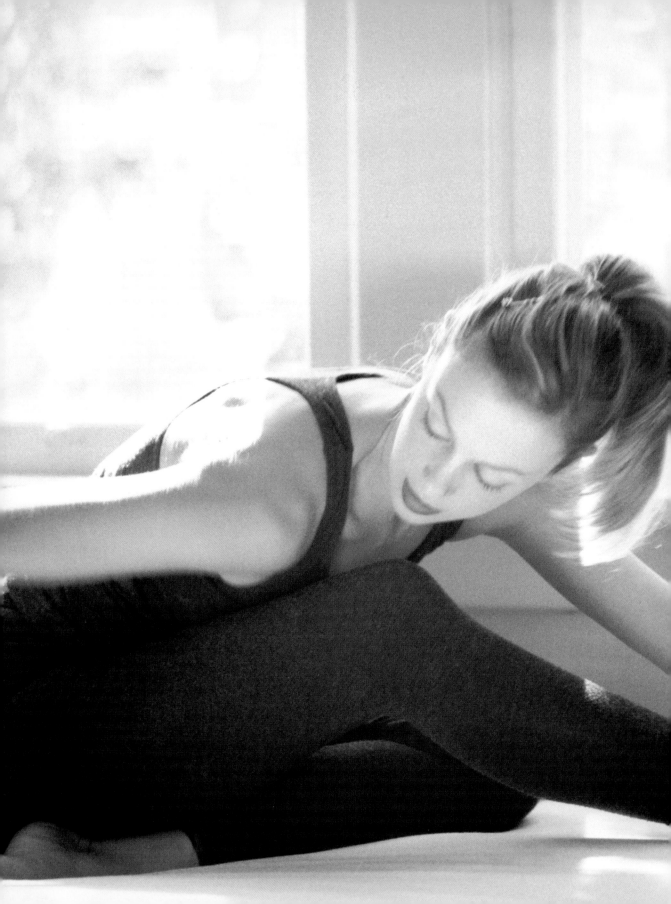

1 WhichBodyTypeAreYou?

For many years, doctors and exercise gurus have divided people up according to whether their natural body shape is slim, curvy or muscular. These three body types are called ectomorphs (slender), endomorphs (rounded) and mesomorphs (muscular). In addition, people are divided into 'apple-shaped' or 'pear-shaped' types, according to where fat tends to accumulate on the body if they gain weight. Identifying your own body type is important – be brave and honest! – because each type has a different metabolic rate as well as different requirements in terms of cardiovascular exercise, muscle-building exercise and stretching to maintain flexibility. It isn't realistic to expect to change from one body type to another, but with the right exercise and an appropriate eating plan you can improve your shape, and by learning to love your shape you can take positive steps to look your best, whatever your body type.

different *body shapes*

Once you have identified your body type, you can start to plan your eating and exercise regime. In addition to following the ten-minute toning programme, it will really help you to do some form of regular cardiovascular exercise, and the descriptions below will help you to identify the most appropriate form of sport for your body type.

Skinny minnies

The classic ectomorph is super thin, with small bones, narrow hips, and long arms and legs. These people have fast metabolisms and their problem is usually with gaining or maintaining weight, rather than with trying to lose it. They are light and flexible, but find it hard to build muscle when they exercise. Most people would envy their slimness and their ability to eat without gaining weight, but many ectomorphs wish they had more curves or better muscle definition.

It is possible for an ectomorph to build muscle. To do so, they need to combine an exercise programme aimed at building muscle with a diet that features extra meals and healthy high-calorie foods. When exercising, ectomorphs will need to focus on weight training if they want to add bulk. At the same time, they should keep up their cardiovascular work and stretching so that they stay fit and flexible. When eating to gain weight, ectomorphs should add extra servings of foods such as lean meat, nuts and

Even slender ectomorphs can have a weight problem – that of trying to gain and maintain weight.

avocados rather than eating foods that are high in sugar or in saturated fat, which is bad for the heart.

Ectomorphs have a natural advantage in many sports. Their light frames and flexibility make them ideally suited to long-distance running, track and field sports, cycling and basketball.

Roly-polys

Endomorphs are, quite literally, on the opposite end of the scale. They have soft, curvaceous bodies and a tendency to gain weight. This can be discouraging and many endomorphs feel that rather than eating chocolate, they might as well apply it directly to their hips! While some ectomorphs probably envy the endomorph's curves, no one envies their shape if they let fat get the upper hand.

To change their shape, endomorphs need to burn fat by exercising and learn to love a low-fat diet. Endomorphs may not metabolise food as quickly as other body types, so they may have to eat fewer calories in order to lose weight or maintain their weight. Luckily exercise can help. Muscle burns more calories than fat, so building

Endomorphs have to be careful not to allow fat to get the better of their natural curves.

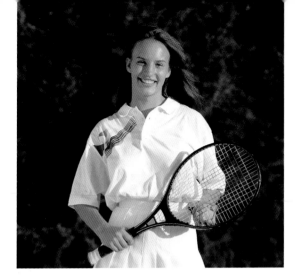

Tennis is an excellent sport for endomorphs, making good use of their strength and their powerful lower bodies.

muscle by exercising regularly will speed up the metabolism, helping even endomorphs slim down.

The good news is that endomorphs are well suited to many sports that will help them keep those sexy curves in trim. They are strong, and have lots of power in their lower bodies. Tennis, weightlifting and martial arts all make good use of those reserves of power.

Mostly muscle

With a strong, muscular build, mesomorphs are the athletic type. They have broad shoulders, big bones and thick muscles. Think of the classic bodybuilder shape, and that's a mesomorph. Even the new slimmed-down Madonna reveals her mesomorph roots – broad shoulders, muscular build, fairly wide waist and narrow hips.

Mesomorphs build muscle easily, but since they have to struggle to maintain flexibility, stretching is essential. Although the mesomorph build sounds like a happy medium, it's not all plain sailing: mesomorphs can gain weight if they don't watch what they eat and they can become muscle-bound if they don't make stretching part of their exercise routine.

Mesomorphs need a balanced exercise regime of weight-training, cardiovascular exercise and stretching to keep their bodies in optimum condition. They are naturally suited to weight work, so they'll need to learn to love stretching (which, if they have let their muscles bulk up too much, will be hard for them) and cardio work (since they usually don't find it fun to run, the rowing machine is a better cardio workout choice).

Learn to love your body type

Everyone is born with a certain predisposition to one of these body types – take a look around your family and you will see others with your shape. Learning to accept and love your body type will make life, eating and exercise more fun. But loving yourself means caring enough about yourself to maintain your health. If your body shape is making you unhealthy because you are way over or under the appropriate weight for your height, do something about it. Similarly, if your lifestyle is making you unhealthy – you never find time for exercise, you get breathless climbing stairs, and you have less energy than you used to – you can do something about that too. Eating right and getting enough exercise will shape up your body, whatever your body type.

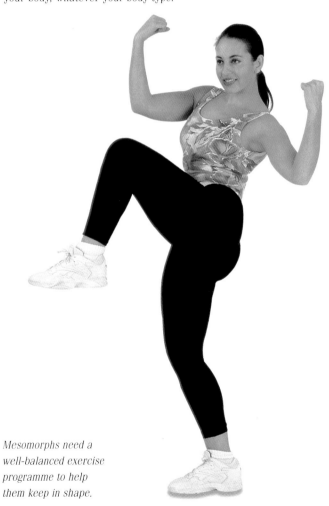

Mesomorphs need a well-balanced exercise programme to help them keep in shape.

are you an *apple* or a *pear?*

Some of us tend to gain weight on our lower bodies, particularly the hips and thighs, while for others a barrel shape comes naturally, with weight gathering around the waist and stomach. Where body fat sits makes a difference to your health as well as your appearance. Research has shown that people with waists larger than their hips have a higher risk of stroke, heart disease, diabetes and cancer.

Apples and pears

Doctors divide people into two types – those who gain weight around the middle, known as apple-shaped, and those who gain weight around the hips, buttocks and thighs, known as pear-shaped. They have found that 'apples' tend to have more health problems while 'pears' have fewer. The tendency to have an apple or pear shape is usually inherited.

Studies have found that people who are barrel-shaped apples and carry fat around the middle (buttocks, belly and abdomen) are more likely to suffer from heart disease, stroke, high blood pressure and diabetes than people who carry their weight around the hips and thighs. Carrying fat around the middle also means that the risk of developing uterine cancer, breast cancer and raised cholesterol levels increases.

The problem with apples

Since apples store their fat in the abdomen, around the internal organs, it is easier for this fat to enter the bloodstream where it can clog the arteries. Fat stored in the middle of the body is stored deeper than fat stored in the lower half of the body. This deep fat seems to cause more fatty acids to be released into the bloodstream, which in turn raises triglyceride and cholesterol levels and makes it harder for insulin to be used in the body, thus increasing the risk of diabetes. All of these factors explain why abdominal fat is particularly hazardous to your health.

It has also been claimed that insulin plays a part in distributing body fat to the upper body. This may be one reason why after people lose weight, they tend to gain it back in the upper body. On the plus side, weight that has been gained last often comes off first. Reducing your weight through diet and exercise may change you from an apple back to a pear, if you were a pear before.

Men are more likely to be apples than pears, while women are more likely to be pears than apples, causing some researchers to believe that sex hormones

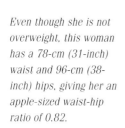

Even though she is not overweight, this woman has a 78-cm (31-inch) waist and 96-cm (38-inch) hips, giving her an apple-sized waist-hip ratio of 0.82.

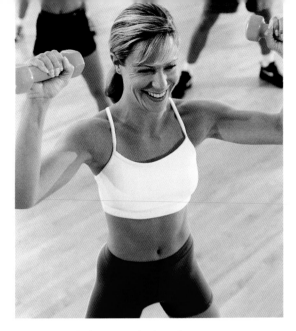

*Taking control of your weight through
healthy eating and regular exercise
can change an apple into a pear.*

and measure your hips at their widest point, then measure your waist. Next, divide your waist measurement by your hip measurement. For women, if the result is under 0.8, you're a pear, but if it is over 0.8, you're an apple. A woman who has a 71-cm (28-inch) waist and 96-cm (38-inch) hips has a waist-hip ratio of 0.74 and is therefore a pear, while a woman who has a 78-cm (31-inch) waist and 96-cm (38-inch) hips has a waist-hip ratio of 0.82 and is an apple. Losing weight and changing your waist-hip ratio can make a big difference to long-term health. A man should have a waist-hip ratio of 1.0 or less, which means that his waist should be the same size or smaller, rather than larger, than his hips.

Changing apples to pears

Although fat stored deep in the abdomen is harder to lose than fat stored on the hips and thighs, it can still be shifted. Losing weight is the best way to change your body shape, and the best way to lose weight is with a combination of diet and exercise. Reducing the number of calories you eat at the same time as increasing your activity level will make you lose weight. Changing to a balanced, healthy diet that is low in fat, but high in vitamins, minerals, carbohydrates and fibre will keep you healthy as you lose weight. If you exercise at the same time, you will get a twofold benefit: you will burn off calories and speed up your metabolism, making the weight come off faster. However, it is best to aim for slow and steady progress – 0.5 kg (1 lb) a week is ideal.

play a part in determining where fat is stored. Some women change from pears to apples after the menopause. If they are also overweight, they are then at higher risk of developing breast cancer.

Waist-to-hip ratio

There is a scientific way to find out if you are an apple or a pear that goes beyond just looking in the mirror. You need to get a measuring tape that doesn't stretch

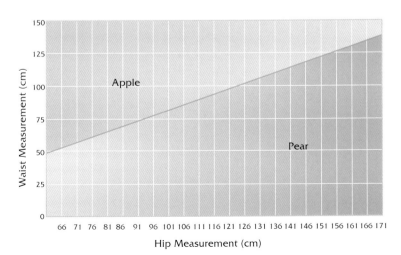

Use this chart to identify your waist-to-hip ratio. This will establish whether you are an apple or a pear.

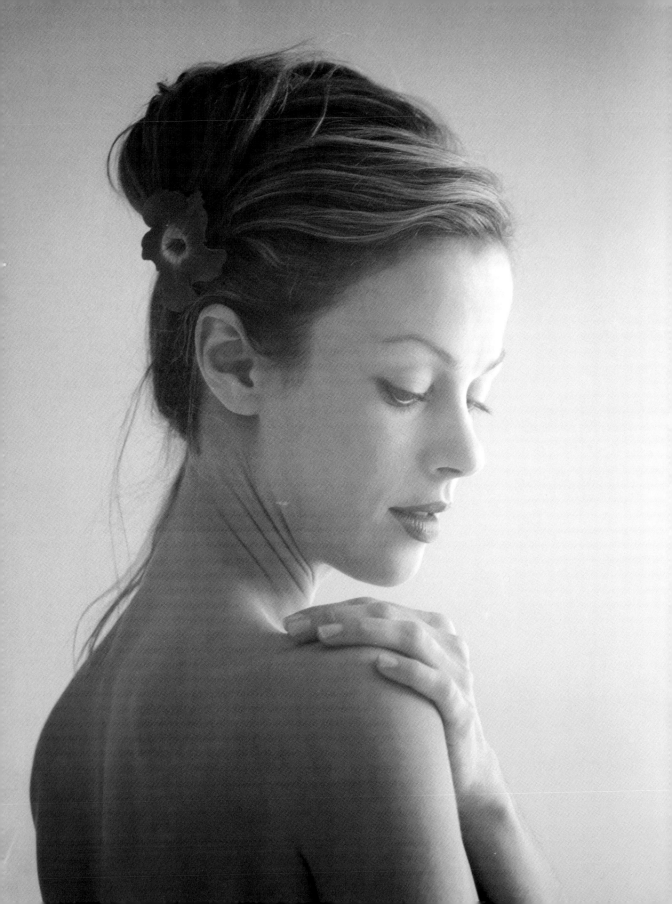

2   BasicAnatomy

Before you start any exercise programme, it is very helpful to have a basic knowledge of the body's structure, just so that you can understand how everything works and how important it is to look after yourself. Put very simply, the skeleton is the framework of the body, and the joints – such as the elbows, hips and knees – allow movement to take place, aided by the muscles. If the joints and muscles are not exercised regularly, they can quickly lose strength and mobility, resulting in pain or injury. The spine has an enormous amount of work to do, especially in the lumbar region of the lower back where big movements such as twisting and bending take place. The lumbar spine is aided by the muscles in the abdomen, so regular practice of the tum exercises will not only improve your appearance but will also have the added benefit of strengthening the muscles that support your back.

the *spine*

The spine is a truly remarkable structure, which is often not treated with the respect it deserves. It holds us upright, but at the same time allows us great flexibility of movement in all directions. If you don't take care of your spine by keeping your weight down and your exercise level up, you will increase the likelihood of suffering from back pain.

The structure of the spine

The spine runs down your back in an S-shaped curve. The 33 bones of the spine – the vertebrae – are stacked one on top of the other. The spine is divided into five sections: the cervical spine, the thoracic spine, the lumbar spine, the sacrum and the coccyx. The vertebrae protect and enclose the delicate spinal cord, which co-ordinates movement and transmits messages between the brain and the body.

The S-shape of the spine is made up of three curves, going in at the cervical spine, out at the thoracic spine, and in again at the lumbar spine. These curves reduce stress on the body, and prevent movement jarring the body – if our backs were literally straight, every step would send a judder up from our feet.

The vertebrae

The seven vertebrae of the cervical spine (neck) support your head. This section of the spine is very flexible, allowing you to tilt your head backward and forward and to look over your shoulders.

The 12 thoracic vertebrae are larger and less flexible than the vertebrae of the cervical spine. The thoracic vertebrae anchor the ribs and hold up the chest, protecting the lungs. Twisting or rotating movements of the upper body are made using this part of the spine.

The five lumbar vertebrae in the lower back are the workhorses of the back. These large, sturdy vertebrae hold up the back and take the strain when we pick up

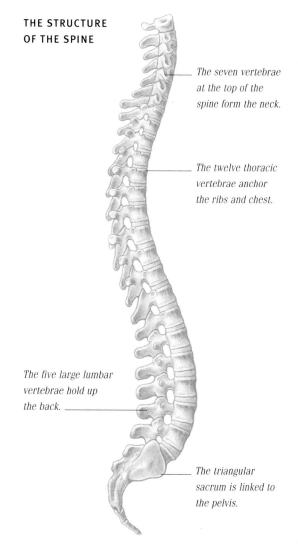

THE STRUCTURE OF THE SPINE

The seven vertebrae at the top of the spine form the neck.

The twelve thoracic vertebrae anchor the ribs and chest.

The five large lumbar vertebrae hold up the back.

The triangular sacrum is linked to the pelvis.

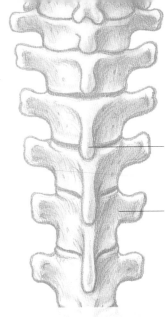

DETAIL OF THE VERTEBRAE

Although the verte-brae are linked, they are very flexible.

Shock-absorbing discs between each vertebra prevent damage.

something heavy, but at the same time they are capable of great flexibility. Because they have to do so much work, they can easily become strained and are therefore the site where back pain is most likely to occur. They are also, along with the cervical vertebrae, the most common place to get arthritis.

At the bottom of the spine is the sacrum, a large triangular bone (or, more accurately, five vertebrae fused together) that is linked to the pelvis by a network of ligaments. The last part of the spine is the tail bone, or coccyx, made up of four small bones that fuse together in adulthood.

The discs

Between the vertebrae are the discs. The discs are made of connective tissues and act like shock absorbers, cushioning the vertebrae. Each disc has a tough outer layer and a gel-filled middle. The discs are incredibly strong; they can bear loads of 1125 kg (2,500 lb). Disc problems are caused either by moving (slipping) or by shrinking. Discs shrink with age, and they shrink during the day owing to the action of gravity. Exercise helps prevent them shrinking.

A slipped disc, also called a herniated or ruptured disc, is a painful problem. The outer surface of the disc may weaken or tear, allowing the gel to leak out to the edges. The unprotected vertebrae then rub together, causing pain, numbness or weakness. Usually doctors advise rest, anti-inflammatory drugs and sometimes

physiotherapy in the hope that the disc will settle down. This treatment is often successful. If the pain continues to be intense, surgery is an option.

Common problems

Back pain is a widespread problem. It is often caused by the combination of a sedentary lifestyle with sudden bursts of activity, such as being desk-bound all week then spending a strenuous weekend gardening or doing DIY chores. The result can be a pulled muscle or a strained lower back. Back pain is also more common the older you get.

Sometimes, however, back pain can be a symptom of a more serious medical problem. You should see a doctor immediately if you have previously had cancer, if you lose control of your bladder or bowels, if you have numbness or weakness in the lower half of your body, or if your back pain is accompanied by fever or unexplained weight loss.

In most cases, however, back pain gets better by itself within one month. You can speed your recovery by resting and reducing the swelling that is causing the pain with ice packs and anti-inflammatory medications for the first few days, followed by heat pads to relax your muscles and the introduction of gentle exercise such as swimming or walking.

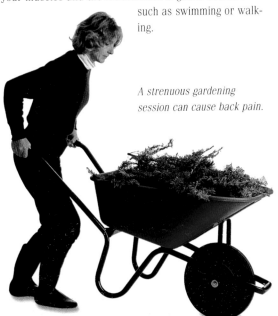

A strenuous gardening session can cause back pain.

the *abdominal muscles*

The abdominal muscles play a key role in protecting your internal organs and supporting your back. The muscles of your abdomen act like a girdle inside your body and run in several different directions across your stomach. You use them when you bend, turn or pick up something heavy. Next time you lift something, pay attention to your body – you will feel your stomach muscles tightening as you lift.

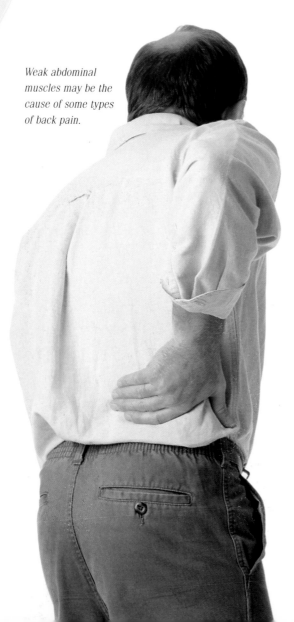

Weak abdominal muscles may be the cause of some types of back pain.

Support your aching back

Once an episode of back pain is over, many doctors advise their patients to strengthen their abdominal muscles by exercising. Building up the muscles of the abdomen and lower back will help make sure that your back pain doesn't recur.

A strong abdomen will help to support the back. The better your muscle tone, the harder your stomach will work and the easier it will be on your back. Having strong abdominal muscles will also improve your posture. Without your abdominal muscles holding your stomach in, swayback (a postural problem where the lower back arches too much, throwing the tummy forward) can occur.

Muscles that move

The muscles of your abdomen allow you to move freely.

The rectus abdominus
This long muscle runs in a vertical line from the ribs to the pubis bone. It contracts to pull your spine forward when you bend forward. It also keeps your chest and abdomen in position.

The rectus abdominus is the home of the 'six pack', that ridged section of stomach muscle that has helped make Brad Pitt famous. Sadly, whether or not you will get a six-pack is down to genetics, not just hard work. Even when they are in great shape, most women and some men have too much subcutaneous fat to show that

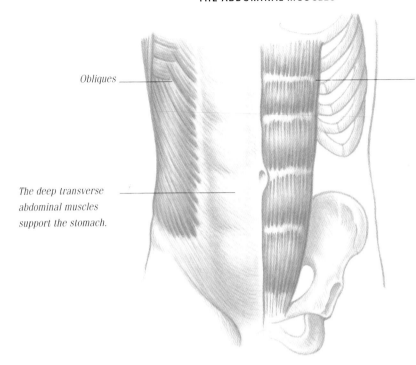

Obliques

The long rectus abdominus muscle contracts to allow the spine to bend forward and to keep the chest and abdomen in position.

The deep transverse abdominal muscles support the stomach.

much muscle definition. So, even though the six-pack is there, you can't see it.

External and internal obliques

These are the muscles of the waist and they run diagonally across the front of your body, allowing you to move forward and back and from side to side. The external obliques are an outer sheet of muscles, running across your body from the ribs to the central rectus abdominus, the pubis and the hips. Underneath, running diagonally in the opposite direction, are the internal obliques. Together, these external and internal muscles form a V-shape across the lower abdomen. As well as protecting your abdomen they help you rotate your trunk.

Deep abdominals

The transverse abdominal muscles support your stomach. This important muscle group forms the deepest layer of your abdominal wall.

Strong, well-toned abdominal muscles mean a firmer, flatter tummy.

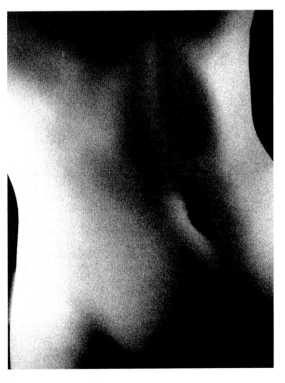

joints

A joint is the connection between two bones, allowing a range of movement from very slight to extreme, such as bending your leg at the knee. Joints, and the fibrous connecting bands called ligaments, allow your body to move with ease, but if you don't take care they can be injured.

Joint types

There are three different kinds of joints: fixed, cartilaginous and synovial. Fixed joints, such as those in the skull, do not move much at all. Cartilaginous joints are semi-rigid but allow some movement. The discs in the back are cartilaginous joints, as is the sacroiliac joint where the sacrum at the base of the spine meets the pelvis. The most mobile of all joints are the synovial joints, which include the fingers, wrists, elbows, shoulders, hips, knees, ankles and toes. These joints have a loose fibrous covering lined with a thin membrane that produces a thick, lubricating, translucent fluid called synovial fluid. This fluid enables the joint to move easily and without friction.

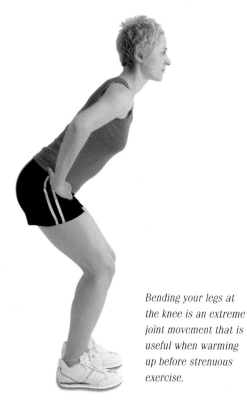

Bending your legs at the knee is an extreme joint movement that is useful when warming up before strenuous exercise.

Joint care

The best way to take care of your joints is to keep them fluid and flexible by exercising and to protect them from sports injuries by warming up properly first. During exercise your joints release synovial fluid, which keeps them flexible. Exercising when your muscles and joints are cold may cause a pulled muscle or an injured joint or ligament. Warming up increases your body's core temperature so that your muscles and joints are loose. Five or ten minutes of marching on the spot, brisk walking or any other gentle activity that makes you breathe faster and break out into a light sweat is sufficient.

Footwork

Some knee or ankle injuries could have been prevented by wearing proper shoes. Many people wear their shoes unevenly, so that one side is worn down before the other. Check to see if you are rolling your feet in or out by standing your shoes at eye level on a flat surface and looking at the backs of the heels: they should be straight.

SYNOVIAL JOINT

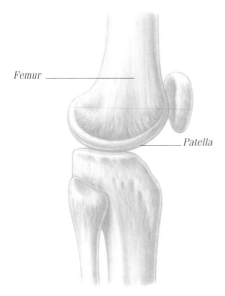

Femur

Patella

Even if you wear your shoes evenly, after a while they will lose their cushioning. Wearing worn trainers makes an injury more likely because the body is jarred or thrown out of balance. Ill-fitting shoes can also cause an injury. If your shoes don't fit properly, replace them.

Some people have flat feet, knock knees or other orthopaedic problems. If these are not corrected, perhaps with specially made shoe inserts, injuries can occur in other parts of the body, particularly the back, hips, knees and ankles.

Ankle supports can help protect your ankles. Ankle-high shoes can be useful if your ankles are weak or if you are doing a sport that is hard on the ankles, such as hiking over rough ground, playing basketball, dancing, playing tennis or playing football.

Ankle injuries can occur when you land badly, rolling over on to the inside of your ankle and pulling the outside. Knee injuries are also common since the knee acts as a hinge, a lever and a shock absorber and sometimes becomes over-strained. Exercise can strengthen the muscles and ligaments around your joints so that they are less likely to be injured.

What to do when it hurts

One thing you should never do when you are injured is try to exercise through the pain. Pain is your body's way of telling you to stop and find out what's wrong! Many muscle and joint injuries can be treated with rest, ice, compression and elevation. If you suspect that you have injured a muscle, ligament or joint, apply an ice pack for 20 minutes every two hours, except when you are asleep, for 48 hours after an injury (if the pain is severe or doesn't get better after 48 hours, see your doctor). You might also want to take an anti-inflammatory medication such as ibuprofen. Elevating the affected area above the level of your heart will reduce the blood flow and therefore the swelling, while bandaging it (compression) will also keep the swelling down. Be sure not to wrap too tightly – if the part of your body farthest from your heart starts to throb (for example your hand, if you have bandaged your arm), loosen the bandage. Try to rest for about 48 hours, then start moving about gradually, but stop if it is still painful. After 48 hours, if there is no swelling, you can apply heat to relax stiff muscles. Hot compresses should be warm, not boiling hot.

Sports injuries are among the most common. It is important to recover fully from injury to avoid permanent damage.

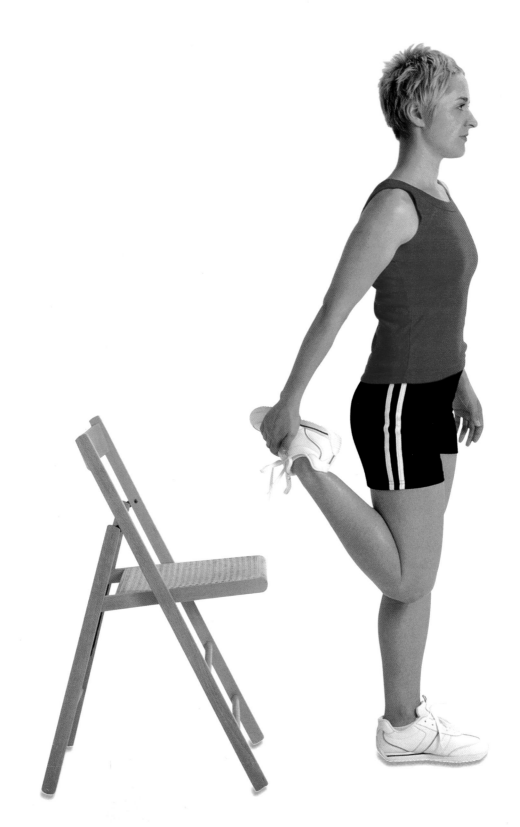

3 Posture

Posture – the way you position yourself when you are standing still, walking or sitting – has a huge impact on many aspects of the body. Poor posture affects your appearance and the way that people perceive you. A stiff, military posture makes a person look rigid and unbending. A slouched posture makes someone look diffident and unsure of themselves. Good posture, on the other hand, projects poise and confidence. Poor posture can cause neck and back pain and may also compress the lungs and abdomen, leading to breathing and digestive problems. Good posture keeps the body in its correct alignment, and allows the internal organs to function efficiently. Unfortunately, poor posture is a habit that many people fall into. The good news, however, is that working the buttocks and abdominal muscles to trim the bum and tum will in turn provide better support for the spine, resulting in greatly improved posture.

what is *good posture?*

Good posture is one of the cornerstones of a fit body and a good appearance. When you are standing straight, you will look and feel more poised and confident, and your back will be under far less strain. In addition, because your body is properly aligned when your posture is correct, you are much less likely to suffer from injuries when you exercise.

Good posture

The correct way to stand is with your head up and centred over your shoulders, your shoulders back and your back flat with a slight hollow in the small of the back. Your hips should be straight, not tilted forward, back or to either side. You can visualise correct posture by imagining that you are a puppet with a string coming out of the top of your head. As the string pulls up, your whole body comes into alignment, one part stacked comfortably over the other. Good posture looks natural and relaxed, neither rigid nor slouched. It also keeps your muscles balanced and toned in relation to one another.

Holding your neck and head in a straight line is part of good posture. If you stick your chin out or habitually tilt your head to one side, perhaps while you are on the phone, your neck has to work harder to hold up the weight of your head – 4–5 kg (10–12 lb). Both of these habits can literally be a pain in the neck.

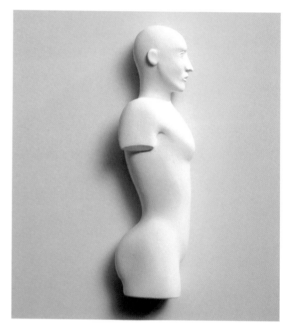

In its correct posture, the back is flat with a slight hollow, and the shoulders are back with the head centred over them.

Bad posture

Although there is only one correct posture, there are many different types of bad posture. Some people have a rigid military stance, with their chins tucked in, shoulders pinned back and chest thrust out, which forces the lower back to arch, straining it. Other people have the opposite problem: they hunch or round their shoulders. This is a popular stance among teenagers and is also common in very tall people and women who think their breasts are too large. Slumping down and rounding your shoulders will not make either you or your breasts shrink, but it can lead to back pain.

Swayback is the term for a lower back that curves inward too much. The lower back should have a slight inward curve, but not a really pronounced one. Arching your back puts a lot of strain on your lower back, and also makes your abdomen stick out, making your tummy look fatter than it is: two good reasons to work on eliminating swayback!

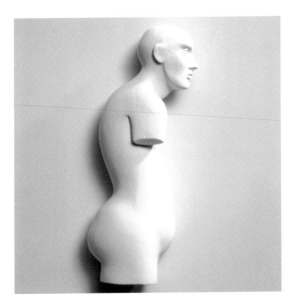

A typical example of poor posture has the shoulders hunched, throwing the head forward and the stomach out.

You should sit up straight with your feet flat on the floor, your knees slightly higher than your hips, and your lower back supported. The desk should be at the right height so that you can fit your chair and your knees beneath it. If you work at a computer, the screen and any paperwork should be at eye level so that you don't need to strain your neck by looking up or down. Your arms should be at right angles to your keyboard. Move the seat of your chair and your back rest up and down until you can achieve the correct position. If you are short, you might need a foot rest or to use a keyboard tray that is lower than the desk top. If you are tall, you may need to have your desk raised up on blocks. Once you are sitting comfortably, remember to get up and stretch once in a while.

Poor posture can actually harm your health, causing back or neck pain and sports injuries. It is the prime suspect in many occurrences of back pain. Getting your posture right by learning what good posture feels like, and by strengthening your back, buttock and abdominal muscles so that you can hold that position effortlessly, can relieve this type of back pain.

Over the years your muscles adapt to poor posture, with some muscles becoming short and tight and the opposing muscles getting longer and slacker to compensate. For example, if your buttocks lack muscle tone, then the opposing muscle group, the hip flexors at the top of the front of your thigh, will have got shorter and tighter. When your muscles become unbalanced in this way, it is easy to injure yourself during exercise because the muscles are not working in harmony.

Are you sitting comfortably?

A lot of us spend our working lives sitting at a desk. The way that we sit can make a big difference to our posture and our health because sitting puts much more strain on the lower back than standing, which is five times more stressful than lying down.

It is important to have your chair at the right height so that your feet can rest flat on the floor.

using muscles for *good posture*

Good posture won't come about just by willing yourself to stand straight and tall. You need to build up muscle power to hold you up in the correct posture so that you can stand properly without having consciously to think about it. The main muscles that influence posture are the buttocks, the hip flexors and the abdominals.

Buttock muscles

The buttocks stabilise the hips, hold the pelvis in the right position and balance the entire hip area. In order to do all that work, they need to be both toned and flexible. If you sit around and don't get any exercise, your buttocks will be slack and lack muscle tone. Even just getting up and walking for 30 minutes a day will improve the muscle tone of your buttocks. Climbing stairs is also helpful. If you work in a building with a lift, try taking the stairs, or getting off at a lower floor, once in a while instead. Doing the exercises in this book will give the muscles in your buttocks an even better workout, of course.

The gluteus maximus is the largest muscle in the body. It is attached to the bottom of the spine at the sacrum and the coccyx, or tail bone, and to the thigh bone. This muscle helps keep your body upright and allows it to rotate at the hips. It also pulls your thighs backward as you walk. Beneath this large muscle are three long muscles, the hamstrings, which run from the back of the hip bone to the back of the knee. They work in concert with the gluteus maximus to bend the knee and pull the legs back as we walk and run.

Hip flexors

The hip flexors are a group of muscles that run from the hip to the lower spine or at various points along the thigh bone. They include the adductor magnus, the adductor longus, and the rectus femoris. They work in

THE BUTTOCK AND THIGH MUSCLES

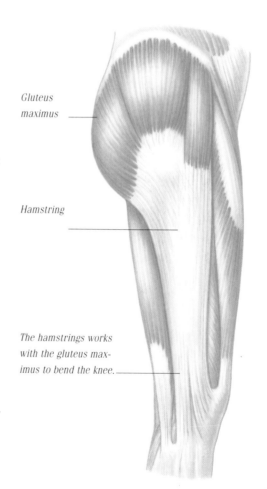

Gluteus maximus

Hamstring

The hamstrings works with the gluteus maximus to bend the knee.

THE HIP FLEXORS

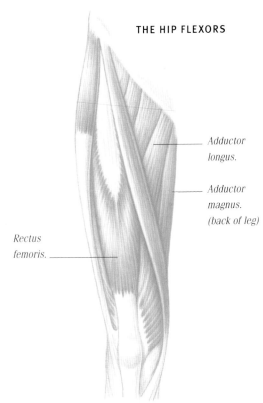

Adductor longus.

Adductor magnus. (back of leg)

Rectus femoris.

Poor muscle tone in the abdomen is usually caused by carrying too much weight or exercising too little. Women who have just had a baby will have poor abdominal muscle tone because their muscles have been stretched during pregnancy. People who have had abdominal surgery will also need to work to get their muscles back into shape.

Poor muscle tone can be corrected with exercise. Many people think that doing sit-ups will improve the muscle tone in their abdomens. Sit-ups can be useful, but they must be done properly so that the abdominal muscles really are doing all the work. The knees should be bent and the hands should never be clasped behind the neck as this may tempt you to haul yourself up. To get the most benefit, come up slowly – if you move too fast, momentum rather than muscle-power is doing a lot of the work. Imagine that the muscles in your abdomen are acting as pulleys, lifting you up. Sit-ups, however, only exercise the external and internal obliques which run from side to side diagonally across the abdomen. These muscles allow you to twist and bend. The muscles that hold your back upright – the transverse abdominal muscles – lie much deeper in the abdomen. They hold your stomach in and support the lower part of your back. To improve your posture, you will need to exercise these muscles specifically (see page 87).

opposition to the buttocks, helping you move your hips, raise your thighs and bring your knees up towards your body as you walk.

If you do a lot of sitting and no exercise, your hip flexors are likely to be tight, while at the same time your buttocks are probably slack and lack tone. The tighter your hip flexors get, the more they pull on the muscles in your buttocks, stretching them and making them even slacker. This is a good example of how a weakness in one part of your body has a knock-on effect, causing a problem in another part of your body. Ideally, both the buttocks and hip flexors would be equally toned and flexible and would therefore exert a balanced pressure on each other. When they get unbalanced, postural problems and sometimes injury result.

Abdominal muscles

The muscles in your abdomen stabilise your lower back and hold your body in alignment. If your abdominal muscles are weak they can't do their job and your back has to do too much of the work, causing lower back pain.

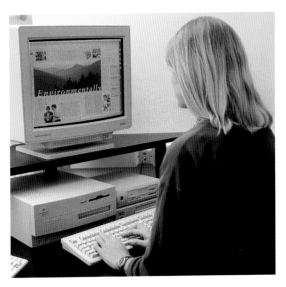

Sitting in the same position for hours on end may lead to a problem of tight hip flexors and slack buttock muscles.

improving your *posture*

Good posture is essential when exercising, both from a safety aspect and if the best results are to be achieved. Good body alignment can influence your body shape and your self-image. By simply standing taller, you can make yourself appear thinner, no matter what your size.

Check your posture

Basically, it's very simple: you must stand straight with your body aligned. Exercise with poor posture and you'll be training your muscles incorrectly.

Stand with your feet hip-width apart, toes facing forward, with your weight evenly distributed. Gently pull up through your legs, keeping your knees slightly bent. Your hips are centred under your shoulders and your pelvis is tilted slightly back. Lengthen your spine, contract your abdominals, sucking your tummy button into the back of the spine as you stand tall. Keep your shoulders down and relaxed, so that your neck is as long as possible. And remember to breathe smoothly!

Practise this standing against a wall. To see that you're doing it correctly, place your hand between the wall and the lower part of your back. If you can get your whole hand through, your pelvis is either tilted too far back or your lower back is too arched. If you can't get your hands through at all, you need to adjust your pelvis – this time it's probably too far forward – and your back is too flat. Ideally, you should be able to place your fingers through the gap.

Now check your posture in a mirror. Standing side-on, with your feet hip-width apart and your knees slightly bent, gently tilt your pelvis forward and backward, then side to side. You need to find a neutral position with a natural curve in your lower back. Your pelvis should not be too far forward or too far back.

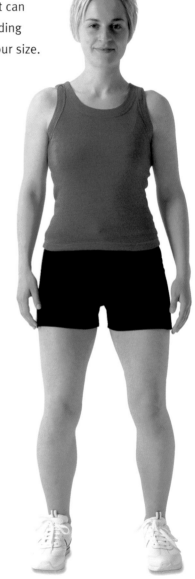

For good body alignment, it is essential to keep your body weight evenly balanced over both feet.

posture
exercises

 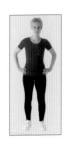

10 MINS

To help maintain good posture not only while working out but throughout the day, too, it's a good idea to exercise the abdominal and buttock muscles to ensure strength and stability of the spine. To work the buttock muscles effectively, you need consciously to contract your abs (abdominal muscles).

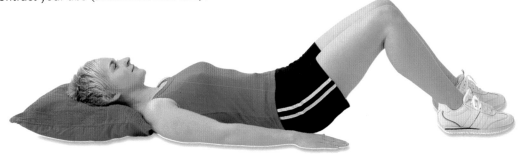

Tummy tightener

- For comfort, lie on a mat and place a cushion under your head.
1 Lie on your back, knees bent, feet slightly apart and firmly on the ground.
2 Starting in the groin area, gently draw in the lower part of your abs and flatten your back to the floor.
3 Hold for a count of two, then release for two, gradually building up to a count of five for each movement.

Remember ...
- *Keep your back flat.*

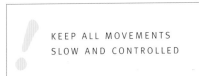

KEEP ALL MOVEMENTS
SLOW AND CONTROLLED

Shoulder rolls

1 Stand tall with your feet hip-width apart, abs in, chest high.
2 Lift your shoulders up and back, then down and forward, in a circular motion.

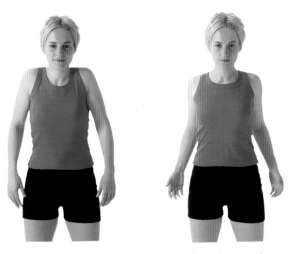

3 Repeat eight times, then reverse the action, starting in a forward direction, eight times.

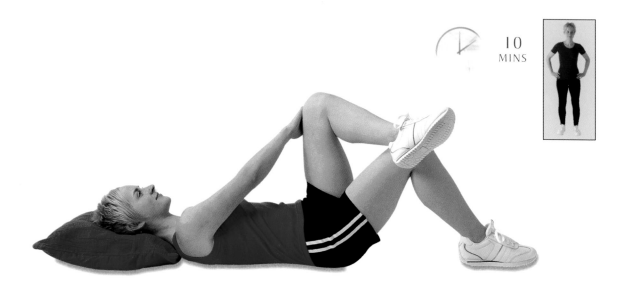

Waist tightener

1 Lie on your back, knees bent, feet slightly apart and firmly on the ground.
2 Gently draw in your abs as for the tummy tightener exercise.
3 Hold the contraction and, as you do so, bring your right hand over to meet your left knee and push your knees slightly against each other.
4 Hold for a count of two, release for two, then repeat on the other side.
5 Gradually build up to one set (8–12 repetitions on each side).

Remember ...
• *Breathe.*
• *Keep your back flat.*
• *Keep your upper body relaxed.*

Buttock tightener

1 Lie on your stomach with your face down.
2 Legs are straight and slightly apart in a V-position, with your knees slightly bent.

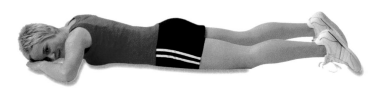

3 Now gently lift one foot a few inches off the floor, then lower.

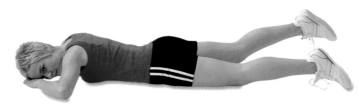

4 Lift and lower for one set (8–12 repetitions) on each leg.

Remember ...
• *Keep your pelvis pressed into the floor.*
• *Keep your abs tight.*
• *Squeeze your buttock muscles.*
• *Don't raise your leg too high.*

Back extensions

1 Lie on your stomach with your face down.

2 Place your hands either by your side with the palms down or resting on your buttocks.

3 Keeping your hips pressed into the floor, use your lower back muscles to lift your chest gently off the floor, then lower.

4 Do one set (8–12 repetitions).

Remember …
• *Try to keep your neck straight and relaxed.*

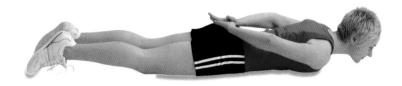

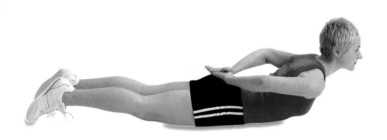

Body balance

1 Kneel on all fours with your knees under your hips and your hands directly under your shoulders.

2 Keep your back flat and contract your abs to support your spine and to help with your balance.

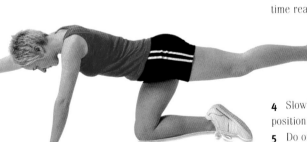

3 Slowly reach forward with one arm and at the same time reach back with the opposite leg.

4 Slowly bring your leg and arm back to the starting position and repeat on the other side.

5 Do one set (8–12 repetitions).

Remember …
• *Pull in your abs.*
• *Keep your pelvis balanced without rotating to one side.*

don't forget to *stretch*

The debate continues as to whether stretching in the warm-up has any real benefits. If you choose to stretch in the warm-up, only do so when the muscles are warm, and always stretch in the cool-down after resistance work or aerobics. As part of the cool-down, when your muscles are warm and more pliable, it is possible to increase the stretch, thereby increasing flexibility.

Quad/front of thigh stretch

1 Stand tall with your feet hip-width apart, knees slightly bent.
2 Using a wall or a chair for support, bring your right leg up behind you and grasp the middle of your foot or heel with your right hand.
3 Gently ease it towards your bottom. Hold for a minimum of 10 seconds.
4 Repeat on your left leg.
5 Feel the stretch in the front of your thigh.

Remember …
• Tilt the hips slightly forward.
• Keep the knees slightly bent.
• Hold the abs in tight.

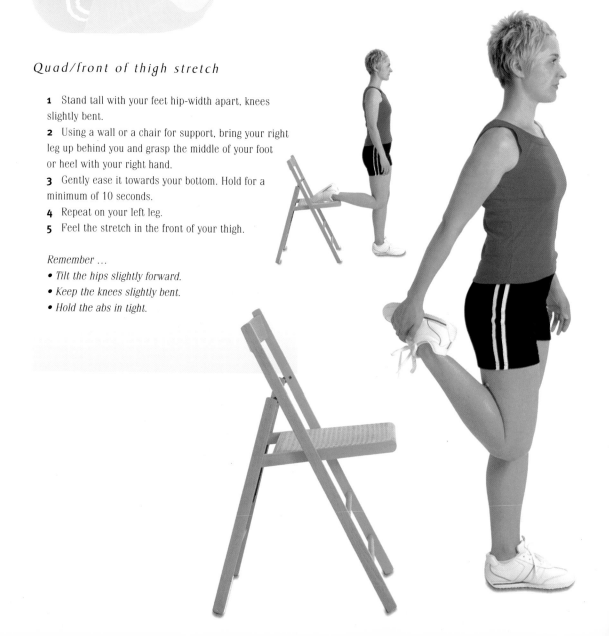

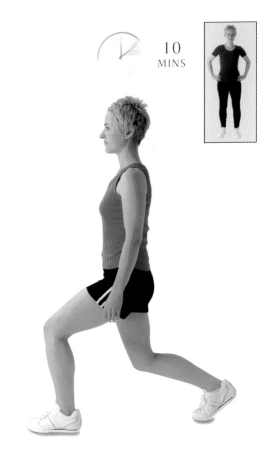

10
MINS

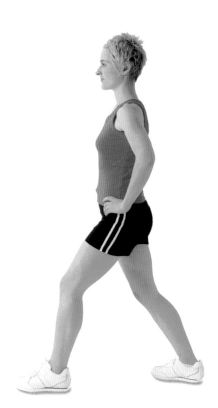

Hip flexor stretch

1 Stand tall with your feet hip-width apart.

2 Step back with your right leg, bend both knees and lift your right heel off the floor.

3 Keep your pelvis tucked under, and hold.

4 Repeat on your left leg.

Remember …
- *Your posture – upper body is upright.*
- *Hips and feet face forward.*
- *Abs are held in tight.*

Remember …
- *The key to a good stretch is to move into each position slowly until you feel a mild tension, then stop.*
- *Hold the stretch and concentrate on how it feels.*
- *Never force your body into a stretch, simply relax into it.*
- *Your breathing technique is very important. Holding your breath will cause tension and strain. Go into each movement on an out breath, then breathe normally.*
- *In the warm-up, hold the stretch for 6–10 seconds; in the cool down, hold for 15–30 seconds.*
- *Come out of a stretch with as much care as you go into it.*
- *Practise your stretches slowly and with concentration – don't bounce!*
- *If, at any point, you feel increased tightness or pain, stop!*

Buttock stretch

1 Lie on your back with your knees bent.

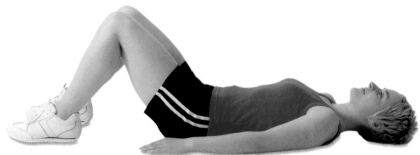

2 Place your right foot on your left knee and lift your left leg off the floor.

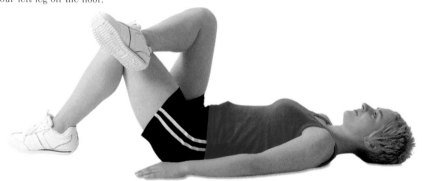

3 Holding your left thigh, gently draw your left knee towards you, pushing your right knee to the side.

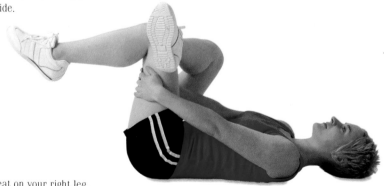

4 Hold, then repeat on your right leg.

Remember …
- *Keep the upper body relaxed.*

Lower back stretch

1 Lie on your back, pull your knees into your chest and bring your arms around them in a hugging position.

2 Gently lift your head off the ground to meet your knees and hold for a minimum of 10 seconds.

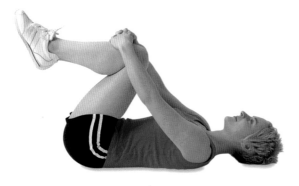

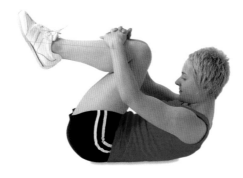

Remember ...
- *Breathe.*
- *Keep your body relaxed.*

Back stretch

1 Lie on your stomach with your elbows bent and your hands flat on the floor in front of you.

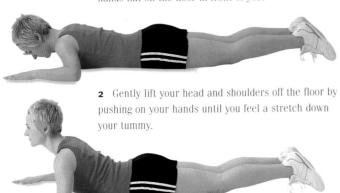

2 Gently lift your head and shoulders off the floor by pushing on your hands until you feel a stretch down your tummy.

3 Hold for 10–30 seconds, then lower.

Remember ...
- *Look straight ahead of you.*
- *Lengthen your spine.*
- *Keep your hips on the floor.*

---

posture programme

Spend about 30 seconds on each exercise on each side (where worked separately).

Warm-ups

1 Shoulder rolls
2 Marching on the spot until you feel warm

Toning exercises

1 Tummy tightener
2 Waist tightener
3 Buttock tightener
4 Back extensions
5 Body balance
6 Stretch
Hold each stretch for 10–30 seconds.
- Quad stretch
- Hip flexor stretch
- Buttock stretch
- Lower back stretch
- Back stretch

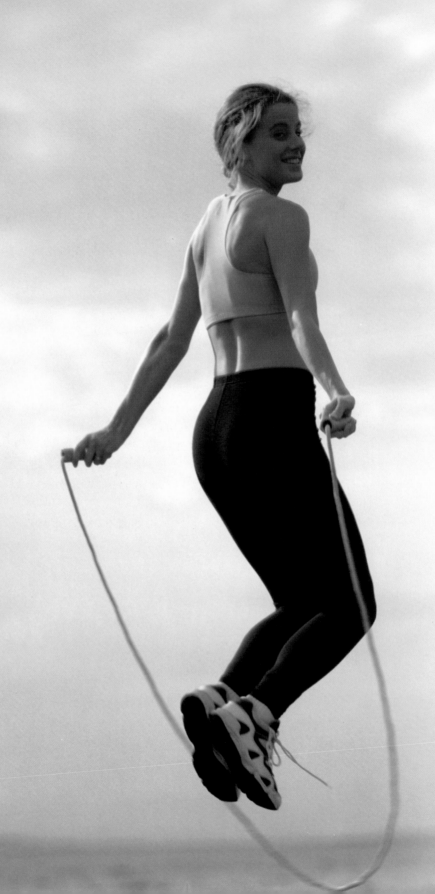

4 AssessingYourFitness

It is very tempting, once you have made the decision to start exercising, to go at it over-enthusiastically – you can't wait to see the results, and the words 'no pain, no gain' dance before your eyes, urging you on. This, however, is definitely not the way to begin – you must work according to your level of fitness. If you have not exercised in a long time, and/or if you are over 45, contact your doctor before starting the programme – a few simple checks will determine your state of physical fitness. You should also talk to your doctor if you already have asthma, heart problems, high blood pressure or arthritis. And even if you do take some form of regular exercise, targeting a particular area of the body may use your muscles in a different way, so it is still necessary to aim for steady progress.

how *fit* are you?

Fitness is made up of four different components: cardiovascular endurance (how strong your heart and lungs are), muscular strength (how hard you can do something), muscular endurance (how often you can repeat an action) and flexibility (the range of movement in your joints). Much of the work in this book focuses on muscular strength and endurance in the abdomen and buttocks.

Take it slow

If you don't take any form of regular exercise, and you have a desk job and don't move about much, then your sedentary lifestyle means that you are probably not very fit. If, on the other hand, you have a job that takes you out and about or you have small children to run after, if you walk everywhere or you play sports regularly, you are probably quite fit.

No matter how fit or unfit you think you are, start with the beginner's exercises. If they are too easy for you, you will soon realise it and can then step up a level until you find the level that is right for you. If even the beginner's level is too difficult, don't get discouraged – just do fewer exercises more slowly, and you will soon find that you are ready to progress. The aim is to exercise at a level that tires your muscles but doesn't leave you exhausted and sore for days afterwards.

Tense up to tone

Exercises aimed at your abdominal muscles and your buttocks are intended to make them more toned, to lift them, to make them firmer and to create a more pleasing shape – lifted and pert for your bottom, flatter and firmer for your stomach. What they will not do is spot reduce fat from one particular area of your body – that is impossible.

In addition to making specific areas of your body look better, these exercises, if done correctly, will also improve your posture and make you stronger. Being

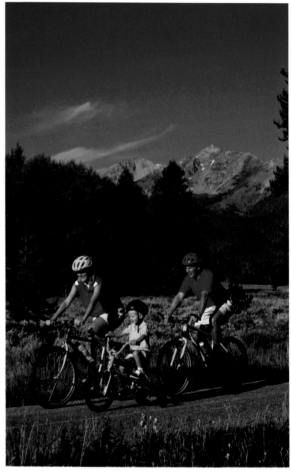

Cardiovascular exercise, such as cycling, keeps you healthy by exercising your heart and lungs, making them stronger.

stronger will give you more energy and make it easier for you to lift shopping and heavy items, or just to enjoy your daily life. Good posture and strong abdominal muscles go hand in hand. They are also two of the best weapons against lower back pain.

The more muscular you are, the faster your metabolism will be because muscle burns more energy than fat. Developing your muscles will actually make it easier to control your weight.

Strength versus endurance

You need to develop your muscles in two different ways: through strength and through endurance. Strength is the force a muscle produces in one burst. Imagine being at a fun-fair and hitting the bell with the hammer – how high the bell goes shows how strong you are. Endurance means doing something over and over again with great force, breaking rocks with a sledge hammer, for example. Each stroke of the hammer is not as hard as when you hit the bell in the fun-fair, but the activity can go on for a long time.

To increase both your strength and your endurance, it is necessary to repeat the exercise until your muscles feel tired. At first you might find that you can only do an exercise three or four times in a row. During the next session, try to do more, always working to your maximum – the most you can do comfortably. Gradually, as your muscles become stronger and your stamina increases, you will be able to do more and the number of repetitions will increase.

How to work your muscles

In order to strengthen your muscles, you need to exercise against some form of resistance. In the gym, weights are used and the muscles are worked against the weights. Gradually, the amount of weight can be increased, making the muscles work harder. Rowing machines also provide resistance to all the major muscle groups.

It is also possible to use your own body to create resistance. Push-ups are a good example of an exercise that uses only body weight to create resistance. The arms push up the weight of the body and in the process

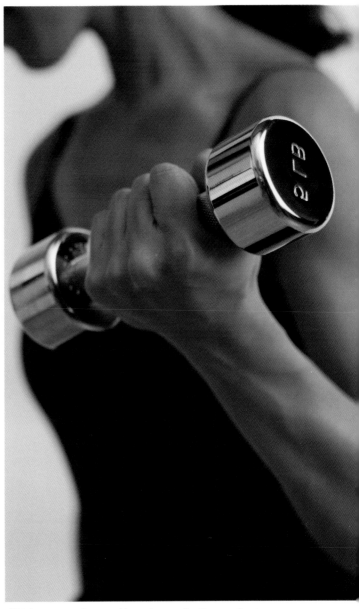

Weights are used to provide resistance for the muscles to work against as you exercise them.

work many different muscles in the arms and chest, and also in the abdomen and buttocks, which must be tensed to hold the body in a straight line during the exercise. Although push-ups are not included in the ten-minute toners, you will be using body weight to create resistance and increase strength.

working out *correctly*

Knowing how to work out correctly will help you to enjoy exercise more. Learning how to warm up and cool down and how and when to stretch will also help you to avoid exercise-related injuries. You should not exercise if you have a cold, flu or other illness. Exercise should not be painful. If you feel any pain, particularly chest or neck pain, stop exercising. If the pain does not go away, see your doctor.

Metabolism and your muscles

Metabolism is the scientific name for the rate at which your muscles burn calories. Different people have different metabolic rates. Metabolic rate may be partly determined by genetics, which is why some people can eat a lot without gaining weight, or do not exercise much but still have nicely defined muscles. How much muscle an individual has also plays an important role in determining metabolic rate because, even at rest,

muscle cells use up energy faster than fat cells. So, the more muscular someone is, the higher will be his or her metabolic rate.

Age and gender also influence metabolic rate. An individual's metabolic rate is quickest at 20 and faster under 30 than over 30. Women, because they usually have less muscle than men, also have a slower metabolic rate. Body size, too, influences metabolic rate. Heavier people use up more calories from performing the same activity – so, for example, a 59-kg (9½-stone) person would use 96 calories in an hour of weeding, while a 82-kg (13-stone) person would use 135 calories.

Muscles that work together

Throughout your body, your muscles work in pairs. As one muscle contracts and pulls part of your body, its opposite relaxes to allow the movement. When you lift your knee upward in a marching step, the muscles at the top of your thigh pull up, while the muscles at the back of your thigh – the hamstrings – relax to allow the movement. Ideally both muscles in a pair should be equally strong, keeping the body in balance. It is more common, however, for the muscles to be unbalanced. If you sit down a lot, the muscles at the front of your thigh are likely to be tight and short, while the muscles at the back will have stretched, becoming longer and slacker, to compensate.

Many muscles in the buttocks and abdomen work in opposition to one another. It is therefore important that you work both sets of muscles to remain in balance.

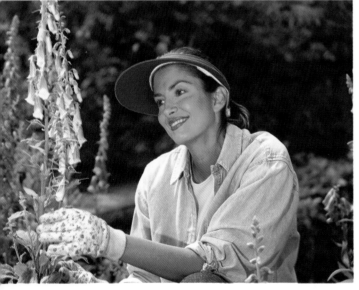

Even gentle weeding burns calories – but how many you use depends on your metabolic rate.

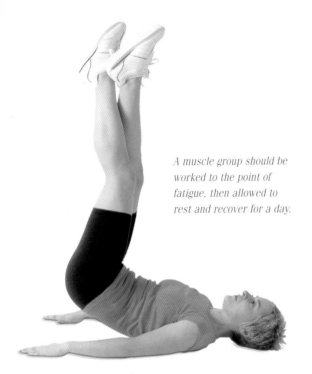

A muscle group should be worked to the point of fatigue, then allowed to rest and recover for a day.

Different muscle groups should be worked on alternate days to give them a chance to rest between workouts.

Toned, not bulked!

Few women, even those who work out regularly, develop bulging muscles. This is because muscle bulk is produced by testosterone, the male sex hormone, and although women have some of this hormone, they do not have enough of it to create big muscles. When women exercise, they usually develop stronger and more toned muscles, not bulkier ones.

Working your muscles

To develop muscle strength, it is necessary to work a muscle group to the point of fatigue, then let it rest and recover for a day, before working the muscles again at their maximum level. With each exercise session, the maximum amount increases slightly and the muscles get stronger and are able to work harder and for longer.

The first stage in muscle strengthening is to overload the muscle. This is done by contracting, or tensing, the muscle against some form of resistance, such as a weight or simply the weight of your body. You should work harder than you would in daily life, and feel some slight muscle soreness for a short time after exercise – if you feel none at all, then you are not working hard enough. If you are so sore that it's painful, however, or the soreness lasts longer than a day, you are overdoing it and need to work a little less hard until you have increased your muscle strength.

As you get stronger, you will need to do more to overload your muscles, either by doing more repetitions in an exercise session, adding more sessions or doing more difficult exercises. This is called challenging your muscles. For these ten-minute toners, the exercises are graded so that you can challenge your muscles by doing harder exercises rather than by devoting more time to exercise.

In exercise, fatigue is the point at which you feel that you cannot go on. To increase endurance, it is necessary to work to the point of fatigue. Your muscles will feel weak and tired, as though they just don't have the energy to do more. Working to this point tells you that you have worked to your maximum exertion. By working to your maximum in every exercise session, you are building strength by making your muscles work harder.

In women, exercise creates muscles that are stronger and more toned – not bigger and bulkier.

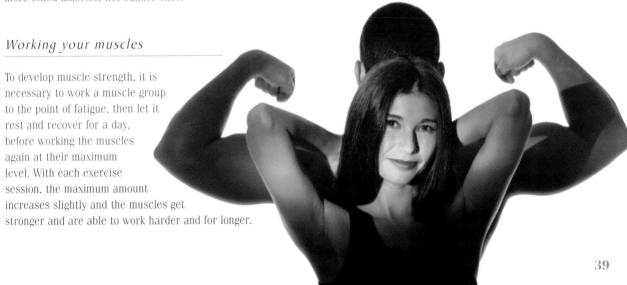

perfecting your *technique*

As you learn new exercise techniques, you are teaching your body new habits. In order to make sure that you are learning the right habits, go slowly, breathe normally and check your position often to make sure you are doing the exercise correctly. Especially in the beginning, doing the exercise the right way is more important than doing it as fast or as hard as possible.

Poetry in motion

When you are exercising, the aim is to be in control of your movements so that you are moving fluidly and smoothly, not in sudden jerks. Although this sounds easy enough, when you are learning new exercises and pushing your body hard, it can be difficult to stay in control of your muscles.

The best way to stay in control is by slowing down. It is more important to do an exercise correctly than to do it quickly. Until you feel comfortable, go slowly, almost as though you are doing the movements in slow motion, and check your position if you are unsure. The aim is to understand how the exercise should feel, so that you get to know when you are doing it right. As your confidence and strength increases, you can stay in control even when you are moving more quickly. That is the time to speed up.

Remember, too, that sudden, jerky movements can cause injury. It is easy to pull a muscle or wrench a joint into the wrong position. Doing an exercise the wrong way, even if it does not cause injury, means that you are not working the intended muscle groups. For example, in many abdominal exercises it is easy to use your thigh muscles or buttock muscles, which are strong, to pull you up, rather than your abdomen, which may lack muscle tone.

Breathing lessons

When you are concentrating on getting something right, it is easy to forget to breathe. Suddenly you realise that you have been holding your breath, so you take in a big gulp of air. If you are not breathing deeply and regularly, you are starving your muscles of the air they need.

As you carry out your exercises, time your breathing to your movements and breathe slowly and deeply. Breathe out through your mouth as you do something that takes effort, such as moving up into a sit-up position, then breathe in through your nose as you lower yourself back down, then out again as you come back up, and so on. Exhaling as you move up has the added benefit of sucking the muscles of your abdomen inward, which ensures that you are working the deep muscles. It also helps to prevent the abdominal muscles 'popping out' instead of tightening up.

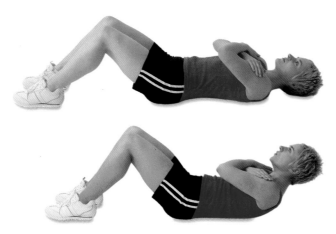

Each movement in an exercise should be fluid and smooth. This will become easier to achieve as you get stronger.

Over and over

Exercises that build muscle are done as a series of repetitions. A repetition is one exercise. A set is a group of repetitions; it usually consists of between six and 15 repetitions. To build strength and endurance, the same exercise is done again and again: one to three sets for each exercise is common. The aim is to work until your muscles feel tired, which strengthens them over time so that they can do more work.

Time out

Muscles need days off to recover from resistance training. The aim of this kind of training is to overload and exhaust your muscles, but working the same muscle group every day is not the most effective way to build strength. By resting them the next day, you are actually helping to build stronger muscles. You can either exercise all your muscles every other day, or exercise every day but working alternate muscle groups. So you might do your abdominal exercises one day, then exercise the muscles of your buttocks the next day. If you have little time, this is the most efficient way to exercise, as you only need a few minutes every day. You should exercise each muscle group three times a week.

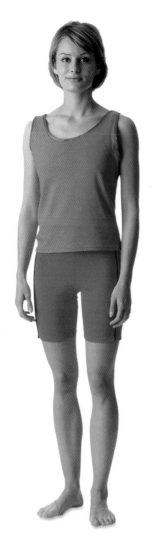

Always check your posture before you start exercising to make sure that your body is in alignment.

Posture perfect

Unless you are standing correctly, you will not be able to do the exercises in this book properly because your hips will be in the wrong position. Take a moment before you start to check that your back is aligned, with your head up, your tummy held tight, your buttocks tucked in and your knees over your feet. If you are not sure that you are standing properly, go to the chapter on posture and do some of the exercises there to remind yourself.

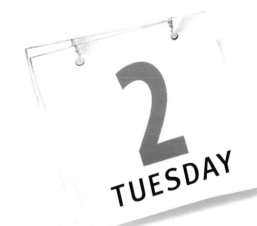

Plan to exercise each muscle group three times a week.

be *flexible!*

The aim of exercise is to build strong, toned muscles – but flexibility is just as important as fitness. Flexibility enables the joints to move through their full range of motion. Stretching after exercise when your muscles are warm increases flexibility by relaxing the muscles and increasing blood flow to the area; over time it lengthens short muscles and allows a greater range of motion.

Flexibility is your friend

Some people are naturally more flexible than others, women are more flexible than men and younger people are more flexible than older people. Within their own limits, however, everyone can benefit from becoming more flexible. And it is never too late: even elderly

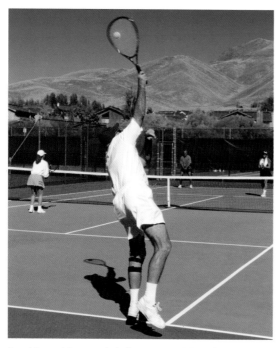

Reaching to hit a tennis ball can cause injury if your muscles are not sufficiently flexible.

people can improve their flexibility. Pregnant women are the one exception to this rule. Pregnancy hormones make the body more flexible in preparation for birth, so over-stretching can cause problems later. Light stretching during pregnancy is fine – just be sure to take it easy (see pages 50–51 for advice on exercising safely before and after the birth).

Being flexible offers protection from muscle pulls and tears that are a common form of injury caused by sudden stretching movements, such as reaching to hit a high tennis ball or even just to swat a fly! Short, tight muscles can easily be overstretched during exercise, so loosening them gradually with gentle stretches can help lengthen them.

Flexibility and exercise

The way to become more flexible is through stretching. The best time to stretch is when your muscles are warm at the end of an exercise session. Stretching at this time has the added benefit of acting as a cool-down. When you finish exercising, it is better to cool down gradually than to stop suddenly. Cooling down may help you to avoid post-exercise stiffness. You can also stretch at the start of a session, after you have warmed up by marching in place, jogging or brisk walking. The one time not to stretch is when your muscles are cold.

Stretching increases flexibility and agility. It is particularly good for people who spend a lot of time sitting down since their muscles are likely to be tense and stiff. Stretching is certainly not just for athletes or gymnasts.

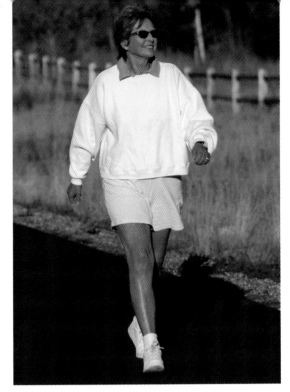

Taking a brisk walk is an excellent way to warm up your muscles before an exercise session.

Easing tight muscles

Becoming more flexible takes time. Short, tight muscles get that way over a long period of time, and they need time to become more supple. Stretching should therefore be done gently and gradually. The stretch should never be painful – the aim is to stretch only until you feel tension. It is a good idea to stretch all the muscles in your body, not just the ones you have been exercising.

Some stretching exercises can cause injury. In addition to stretching when your muscles are cold, it is also dangerous to overflex your joints, particularly the knee or elbow, to overarch your back or neck, to do sudden twisting motions, to bounce during a stretch or to stretch when your body is out of alignment. All of these movements can cause injury because they force some part of your body to stretch in an awkward direction or to stretch too far. Doing stretches quickly, particularly when your muscles are cold, is a sure way to cause problems.

There are two kinds of stretching: ballistic stretching and static stretching. In a ballistic stretch, you stretch to your limit and then bounce. This kind of stretching is rarely recommended because it shortens rather than lengthens muscles and can increase the chance of an injury such as a muscle tear. Ballistic stretching also makes you feel stiff.

The right way to stretch

Static stretching is much better for you and carries little risk of injury. It lengthens and relaxes your muscles, loosening them without causing muscle strain. During a static stretch, the aim is to stretch gradually until your muscles feel resistance. You will feel as though you can't stretch any further. When you reach that point, hold the stretch for a few seconds – try to count at least to three, but you can stretch for a count of up to 30. At this point, you can either reach and stretch a little further, or relax. You can then repeat the stretch. Some studies have shown that stretching after exercise can help remove lactic acid, the by-product of exercise that causes that stiff painful feeling the next day. Even if stretching after exercise doesn't ease stiffness, it will make you more supple and it feels so good that you'll want to keep doing it.

Regular stretching helps to keep you supple.

aerobic *exercise*

The exercises demonstrated in this programme are toning exercises, designed to condition and improve specific body parts – in this case, the bum and tum. For an effective, all-round workout, they should be combined with moderately intense cardiovascular activity or aerobic exercise. Simply put, this means exercising with air or, rather, oxygen.

Muscles also need oxygen in order to function efficiently, and the harder we work them, the more their need increases. As we exercise, our breathing becomes quicker and our pulse rate rises. With continued exercise, muscles soon start to adapt to the workloads they are carrying, and they become more efficient at extracting the oxygen they need. Gradually, they become more toned, you begin to burn fat more efficiently, your heartbeat becomes slower and stronger, and you become fitter.

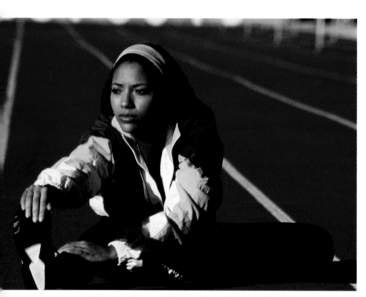

Running is a good form of aerobic exercise. Stretching exercises will warm up the muscles before you start.

Aerobic benefits

Aerobic exercise is any activity that uses the large muscles of the legs and body for a sustained period of time at a speed that increases the body's demand – or, more specifically, the demand of the heart and lungs – for oxygen. It will involve getting hot, sweaty and slightly out of breath. Carried out regularly over a period of time, any form of aerobic exercise will strengthen the cardiovascular system – the heart, lungs and blood vessels – and greatly increase stamina.

Take *five*

1 *Choose aerobic activities that you like.*

2 *Pace yourself – don't rush into anything – and gradually increase the amount of time you work out aerobically.*

3 *Try to exercise aerobically three to five times per week, aiming to do a minimum of 20–30 minutes in each session; break up the sessions if you don't have time to fit in a session this long.*

4 *Don't attempt anything that proves painful.*

5 *If you need to rest, slow down and reduce the pace gradually – don't stop suddenly. If you do, you'll feel dizzy and disorientated.*

There are many activities that give you an aerobic workout. These include brisk walking, hiking, jogging, running, cycling, rowing, step and aerobic classes, swimming and racket sports. When starting out on an aerobic exercise programme, you have to pick something that you enjoy and are capable of doing. It's no good choosing an activity that you don't like and can't do because you won't stick with it for very long, and to gain any benefits from aerobic exercise, it must be performed regularly. The recommendation is to exercise at least three times per week for 20–30 minutes (excluding the warm-up and cool-down). The whole point of aerobic exercise is to do a sequence of movements for at least 20–30 minutes at a steady, rhythmic pace without stopping completely. If you don't have time to fit in a session of this length, then break it down into two sessions. Even a 10-minute workout every day can be of benefit.

Some of the benefits of regular aerobic exercise are:
- An improvement in your breathing.
- Your lungs will get more oxygen, so their ability to clear out toxic waste will be increased.
- Firm and strengthened muscles.
- Improved flexibility.
- A change in your body shape, owing to the redistribution of inches.

All in all, you'll feel better, fitter and healthier. And while aerobic exercise alone won't make you lose weight, it will help you to burn calories. Only by following a sensible eating plan and exercising vigorously on a regular basis will you be successful at losing weight.

Controlling body weight

What woman, at some point in her life, hasn't wanted to lose weight? We seem to be obsessed by diets and our quest to shed a few pounds – or stone! But instead of worrying about how much we actually weigh, we should be concentrating on the amount of fat we have on our bodies. Our body weight is made up of bones, muscles, organs, fluids and fat, and is affected by our height and our build. Muscle weighs more than fat, so a woman who has worked out at the gym and who has strong, toned muscles is more likely to be heavier than a woman of the same build and height who has not.

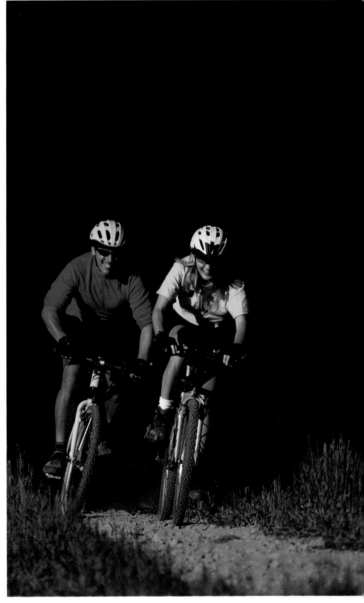

When out on a cycle ride, work hard and rhythmically for about 20–30 minutes for maximum aerobic benefit.

But when we step on the bathroom scales, we're not getting a reading of 'fat' as such, because scales cannot differentiate between fat mass and the rest of our body make-up. And while body weight is often assessed by height-to-weight charts, this doesn't take body composition into consideration.

body mass *index*

The best way to work out your ideal body weight is to work out your body mass index (BMI). This is used to assess your body weight in relation to your height. It is closely related to your body fat percentage. Calculate your BMI using the simple formula below, then check the appropriate range in the guide to see whether you are underweight, the normal weight for your height, or overweight.

$$BMI = \frac{Weight\ (kgs)}{Height\ (m)^2}$$

Calculate your BMI

Working in metric, divide your weight in kilograms by the square of your height.

For example, Weight = 65kg
                Height = 1.65 x 1.65 =2.72
                BMI = 24
                (65 ÷ 2.72)

BMI under 19
Underweight. No need to lose weight, and you may need to gain a little weight if your BMI is significantly below 19. Consult your doctor if you are in doubt.

BMI 19–25
Normal. Aim to keep your weight at this level. You're within healthy guidelines and the risk of weight-related health problems is minimal.

BMI 25–29
Overweight. You are in the 'caution zone'. Your weight should not increase, and it's advisable to lose weight. There is a slightly increased risk of health problems.

BMI 30–40
Officially obese. Reducing weight is highly recommended. The risk of weight-related health problems is increased.

BMI over 40
Very important to lose weight. There is a high risk of early death and weight-related health problems.

Measure your waist

Another way to check whether you are at any health risk because of your weight is by measuring your waist circumference. Place the tape measure loosely around your waist, just above your tummy button.

- Waist circumference below 80cm (31.5in) is classified as healthy.
- Waist circumference over 80cm (31.5in) indicates a slight health risk.
- Waist circumference over 88cm (34.5in) indicates a major health risk.

Using a tape measure is also a good way to monitor your efforts to lose inches from your bum and tum. Before you start on the programme, take one measurement across the level of your tummy button, and another around your hips, at the maximum protrusion of your bottom. Check the measurements at six- to eight-week intervals.

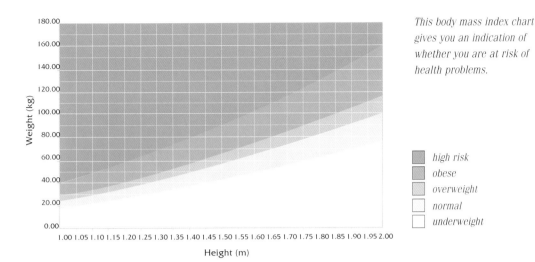

This body mass index chart gives you an indication of whether you are at risk of health problems.

Weight (kg): 180.00, 160.00, 140.00, 120.00, 100.00, 80.00, 60.00, 40.00, 20.00, 0.00

Height (m): 1.00 1.05 1.10 1.15 1.20 1.25 1.30 1.35 1.40 1.45 1.50 1.55 1.60 1.65 1.70 1.75 1.80 1.85 1.90 1.95 2.00

- high risk
- obese
- overweight
- normal
- underweight

Fat

We all need a certain amount of fat to survive. It gives us shape, warmth and insulation, protects our internal organs and provides us with a reserve fuel supply. The problems arise when we store too much fat in the body from overeating and underactivity. The only way to lose it is through burning calories and eating sensibly. The fat cells don't disappear completely, but the amount of fat stored can increase/decrease depending on how well we eat and how much exercise we take.

Cellulite

Most women are familiar with what cellulite is – recent research revealed that more than 95 per cent of women over the age of 35 have it. It's that dimpled 'orange peel' skin that appears on women's thighs and buttocks. And it's not only fat women who get it – being thin is no sure-fire defence. Only men are rarely affected, because the structure of cellulite is hormonally controlled.

Women naturally need more fat around the stomach, hips, thighs and buttocks – without this, they wouldn't be able to sustain a pregnancy. Around every fat cell is a collagen support structure that keeps it together. In men, this particular structure is stronger because of the male sex hormone, testosterone. In women, the support structure is weaker and the cells pucker, producing an unsightly, dimpled effect – cellulite!

An inactive lifestyle contributes to the formation of fat and in women this often appears as cellulite in the legs. Diet is one of the most important factors in treating cellulite. Regular exercise is another – walking briskly, jogging/running, cycling and step or aerobic classes are ideal, as these burn lots of energy, the legs are toned and all the muscles are tightened. While swimming is an excellent form of exercise for burning fat, it's not so good for dealing with cellulite, as the body weight is supported while you're working out in the water. As with any aerobic exercise, to get the best result you need to work out for 20–30 minutes, three to five times a week.

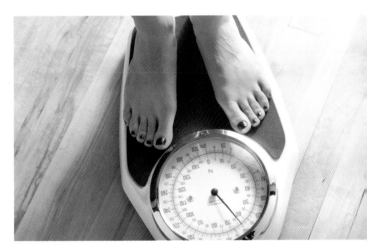

Your weight on the scales may not be the best indication of how fit you are – muscle weighs more than fat.

Assessing Your Fitness   47

burning *calories*

To burn calories, you simply have to boost your metabolism. This is where you need to work out aerobically. Get your heart and lungs to work harder and you will generate more oxygen for use in fat metabolism. The harder and longer you work, the more fat you burn. Continue regularly over a long period of time and your body will become more efficient at burning calories and processing oxygen.

Metabolism boosters

- Try to work out aerobically at least three to five times a week, for at least 20–30 minutes at a time.
- Split the sessions up if necessary – just 10 minutes a day can reap benefits, too.

Roller skating is a fun, energetic outdoor aerobic activity.

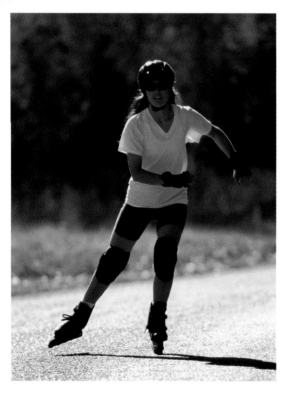

10-minute metabolism boosters for the bum and tum

Keep the movements slow and controlled.

1 Step up and down on the stairs.

2 Now, as you step up, take the other leg out to the side and squeeze your buttock muscles. This is a good one for your outer thigh, but, as you do it, make sure you work from the hip and keep your toes, knees and hips facing forward.

3 To work the buttock muscles, step up and take the other leg out to the back.

Remember . . . Step softly and keep your foot facing forward. Don't arch your back and, as always, keep your abs tight.

There are also small things that you can do in your day-to-day activities that will get you moving. For example, where possible, take the stairs instead of the lift when you're in the office. Walk to the shops instead of driving, and if you have to take a bus, get off one stop earlier and walk the rest of the way. At lunchtime, instead of sitting around after you've eaten, go outside and enjoy a 10–20 minute walk, at a good pace. Even housework can give you a good aerobic workout, if you go at it with some gusto!

Overload

With all exercise, it's important to work at the correct intensity, especially if you're trying to lose weight or get fitter. If you put too little effort into your workout, you'll only get minimal results; if, on the other hand, you put in too much effort, or you work too quickly, this could result in you being injured.

When you 'overload' your muscles, you work them harder than you would during your normal daily activities, especially if you live a fairly sedentary existence. By applying progressive force to stimulate your muscles, you strengthen and tone them. As this happens, they take longer to tire, enabling you to recover more quickly between one exercise and the next.

The aim in any toning programme is to challenge your muscles so that they work harder. This can be achieved in a number of ways: by exercising for a longer period of time, by increasing the intensity of your workout or by increasing the number of days you exercise during the week.

One good thing about a ten-minute toning programme is that you can spend the limited time that you have focusing on just one muscle group. And while it's okay to do different aerobic activities every day, it's not such a good idea to work the same muscle group two days running. This is because the muscles need time to recover fully from a workout. As you perform the exercises, it also helps to rest between each set of repetitions so that the muscles can have a moment to relax and return to their original length.

Fatigue

Your muscles will start to become fatigued during the last repetitions of any exercise. At this point, you may find it difficult to perform another repetition, or your muscles may feel weak and lacking in energy. When this happens, try to do a few more repetitions, even though you are feeling tired, before you stop to take a rest. You may get a burning sensation in the area that you're working, but don't worry – this is normal. As soon as you stop exercising, it will go away.

If you're new to exercise, and, in particular, to exercising your abdominal and buttock muscles, you might find that some of your muscles fatigue more quickly than

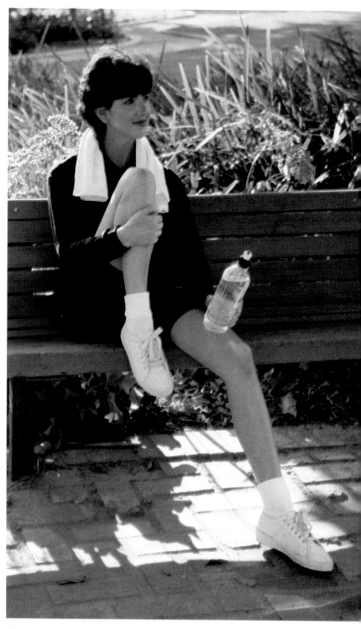

Resting between exercises helps the muscles to relax and to return to their original length.

others. Muscle soreness is fairly inevitable in the beginning, but if you're so sore and stiff that you can hardly move, then you've probably overdone it. Slow down and work at a level that is comfortable but still a challenge until you are feeling stronger.

pregnancy

As long as you are fit and able, it is very important to continue exercising during pregnancy. Obviously, you should not overdo it or perform any movements that may cause stress to the baby or yourself. But certain exercises will help to strengthen the abdominal wall, which is naturally weakened by the developing foetus. And exercise will get you back into shape after the birth.

During pregnancy

Aside from weight gain, the body undergoes some dramatic changes during pregnancy. Ligaments stretch, making the body more flexible, and some joints become more mobile to allow for the growing foetus. The baby's weight changes your posture and you begin to lean back. Carrying a baby puts a lot of pressure on the abs, pelvic floor and spine, particularly around the lower back.

It is important, during and after pregnancy, to exercise the pelvic floor muscles, which support the bladder, rectum and womb. Do this exercise several times a day: close your back passage and your front passage, then pull your vagina in and up in a gripping movement. Aim to hold for 10 seconds or more, resting for 4–5 seconds between each contraction.

Take *five*

1 *Don't gain too much weight in the early stages of pregnancy.*
2 *Eat a healthy, low-fat diet that includes at least five servings of fresh fruit and vegetables a day.*
3 *Keep physically active and exercise, if possible (check with your doctor).*
4 *Spend time stretching ligaments and muscles in preparation for the birth and to strengthen muscles under stress in pregnancy.*
5 *Stop smoking completely.*

Tummy tightener

1 Sit tall on the edge of a chair, feet apart.
2 Place one hand on your stomach, the other on your lower back.
3 Pull your tummy in to tighten your abdominal muscles. Hold for a count of two, then gently release.

Remember …
• *Breathe.*
• *Maintain good posture – don't slouch.*

NOTE: This exercise can also be done standing or lying down.

Waist tightener

1 Kneel on all fours as above right. Pull the baby in towards your spine and gently tilt the pelvis to the right side.
2 At the same time, turn to look over your right shoulder so that your ribs move towards the top of the pelvis.
3 Return to the centre position and repeat on the other side.

Remember …
• *Breathe.*
• *The movement should be slow and controlled.*
• *Only the head, ribs and pelvis move.*

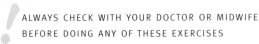
ALWAYS CHECK WITH YOUR DOCTOR OR MIDWIFE BEFORE DOING ANY OF THESE EXERCISES

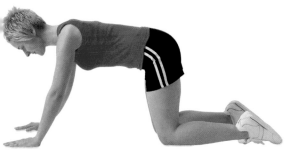

Pelvic tilt

1 Kneel on all fours with your back straight, hands directly under your shoulders and knees under your hips.

2 Gently tilt your pelvis back towards your heels.

3 Tighten your lower abs upward and in, to draw the baby in toward your spine.

4 Hold for a count of two, then slowly relax. Repeat as often as is comfortable.

Remember ...
- *Lengthen your spine.*
- *Don't arch your back.*

NOTE: This exercise is ideal for strengthening your abs. It can also be done standing, sitting, or lying on your back – simply curl or tilt your pelvis forward and backward.

After the birth

During pregnancy, the two sides of the abdominal corset may split apart, leaving a gap. For most women, the muscles will begin to join together a few days after the birth; for others the abdomen may remain distended. To restore your abdominals to good condition, continue doing the antenatal exercises and add those below. Remember to take things slowly – as you become stronger, you can increase the intensity of the exercises and the number of repetitions.

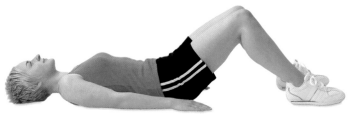

Pelvic tilt

1 Lie on your back with your knees bent, feet placed comfortably apart on the floor, hands by your side.

2 Gently tilt your pelvis forward and hold for a count of four, then relax. Repeat, gradually increasing the number of repetitions as you become stronger.

Curl-up

1 Lie on your back as above with a pillow behind your head. Pull in your tummy.

2 Gently raise your head and shoulders off the pillow, reaching slightly forward with your hands towards your knees.

3 Hold for a count of one, then slowly lower. Relax and repeat, gradually increasing the number of repetitions as you become stronger.

Remember ...
- *Your abs remain flat.*

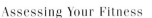

Assessing Your Fitness   **51**

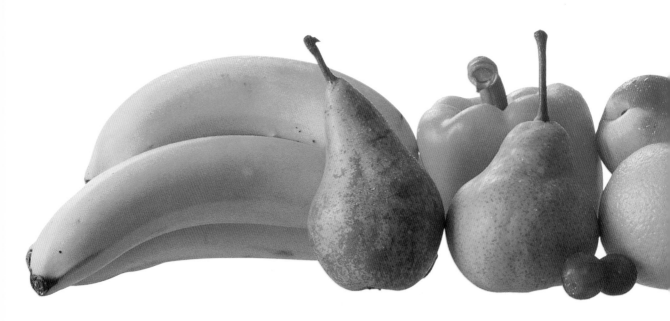

Ten-Minute Toning for Bums & Tums

5 EatingProperly

Eating well is one of the most important things that you can do to stay healthy. A healthy diet includes lots of fresh fruit and vegetables, complex carbohydrates (wholewheat bread, potatoes, grains and cereals, and pulses such as beans and lentils) and a little protein (fish, lean meat and low-fat dairy products). Sugar and fats such as oils, butter and full-fat dairy products should be eaten strictly in moderation, as should highly processed or refined foods. It is all too easy to eat too many fatty and sugary foods, sometimes without even realising it. Unfortunately, eating properly seems to take up far more time than popping a convenience meal in the microwave, so most of us are inclined to settle for a less than perfect diet. However, the benefits of eating well are so great that it's well worth putting some effort into making any necessary changes.

the *basics*

There seems to be endless conflicting advice on what you should and shouldn't eat, depending on whether you specifically want to lose weight, reduce your cholesterol levels, improve the condition of your skin, combat an allergy or for one of many other reasons. When you look closely, however, you will see that the advice is always basically the same – eat plenty of unrefined, natural foods.

The dangers of a bad diet

Studies have linked poor diet to conditions such as heart disease, poor circulation and high blood pressure. The problem foods are those that are high in fat, sugar and salt, leading to excessive weight gain. These substances may be 'hidden' in packaged foods, so always check the labels for ingredients and nutritional information.

Carrying excess weight also puts a strain on the back and joints, and overweight people are more prone to diabetes, stroke, gout, osteoarthritis, digestive disorders and gall-bladder disease, as well as certain types of cancer, particularly cancer of the colon and rectum, prostate cancer in men, and breast, cervical and uterine cancer in women.

The benefits of healthy eating

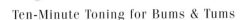

The secret to a healthy diet is simple – eat very little fat and sugar and instead go for lots of fruit, vegetables and wholegrains, as well as some fish, lean meat and low-fat dairy products. These foods are full of nutrients, including antioxidants in the form of beta-carotene and vitamins D and E, which may help prevent the cell damage that

Lean chicken is very low in fat.

can lead to cancer. With this sort of diet, you are unlikely to have a weight problem. You will also be getting plenty of vitamins and minerals without needing to take supplements. You will have clear arteries, normal blood pressure, a healthy digestive system, glowing skin and shining eyes and hair – in short, you will be giving your body everything it needs to be full of health and energy.

Good enough to eat

Nutritionists recommend that you eat plenty of carbohydrates, not very much protein and very little fat. The proportion of calories per day from each group should be: 55% from carbohydrates, 15% from protein and less than 30% from fat. The carbohydrates should come from eating 6–11 servings of starchy foods, 3–5 servings of fruit and 2–4 servings of vegetables. For the protein, you will need 2–3 servings of milk, cheese or yogurt plus 2–3 servings of meat, poultry, fish, dried beans, eggs or nuts. Proteins contain fat and fat is dense in calories, so add extra fat and oil sparingly.

The carbohydrate story

Carbohydrates are starchy or sweet foods, and come in two forms – complex and simple. During digestion, both types are broken down into glucose to provide your body with energy. However, they are not equally healthy – some come naturally packaged with other good things such as vitamins, minerals and fibre, while others don't.

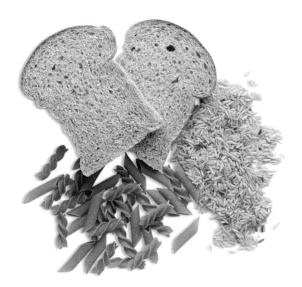

Unrefined foods provide essential nutrients.

giving you a short-lived burst of energy. Fruits contain simple sugars too, but they also contain vitamins and minerals, and fibre in the form of seeds, pulp and skin.

Refined carbohydrates

Some carbohydrates, such as rice and wheat, are refined by removing the hull from the grain, and unfortunately many nutrients and most of the fibre are lost in the process. Many foods, including pasta, breads and baked goods, are made with refined white flour. Wholegrain cereals and breads and wholewheat pasta and brown rice contain more vitamins and minerals and a lot more fibre.

Complex carbohydrates

Carbohydrates such as grains (rice, wheat and oats), pulses (like lentils and chickpeas) and some vegetables (including potatoes and corn) are complex. Bread, cereals and pasta made from unrefined grains are also complex carbohydrates. The process of turning complex carbohydrates into glucose takes time, so the energy made from these foods is released slowly. Complex carbohydrates contain many different vitamins and minerals and some proteins, providing your body with essential nutrients.

Fibre

Fibre – the indigestible part of plants – is very good for your digestive system. A diet high in fibre helps prevent constipation and related problems such as piles and diverticulitis, and possibly cancer of the colon. Soluble fibre, found in legumes, seeds, fruit, some vegetables, oats, barley, brown rice and rye, also binds with cholesterol and removes it from the body, reducing the risk of furred-up arteries.

Simple sugars

Table sugar and products made from it – cakes, biscuits and sweets – are simple sugars. They contain calories but little nutrition, so are often called empty calories. Honey is also a simple sugar. Simple sugars are processed quickly by the digestive system,

Protein

Fish is an excellent source of protein.

Meat, dairy products, fish and eggs all contain protein, as do grains, legumes, nuts and seeds. Proteins are made up of chains of amino acids. Of the 20 different amino acids, the body can make 11: the rest come from the protein in foods. These essential amino acids are found in a complete form in animal products. They are incomplete in vegetable products, but by combining vegetable proteins, such as rice and beans, your body can create a complete protein.

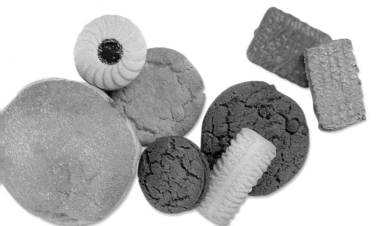

Most biscuits have little nutritional value.

eating in *moderation*

The old saying 'everything in moderation' holds true when it comes to eating. Even fat, with its bad reputation, is an essential part of the diet – as long as you don't have too much. Balance is very important – if you eat a diet that is very high in a healthy food such as fish, for example, but has little in the way of carbohydrates, fruits and vegetables, you are still eating an unbalanced diet.

Fat

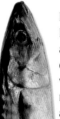

Fat – in small quantities – is good for you. Fats are a high energy food and have twice as many calories per gram (9) as proteins or carbohydrates (4). Young children need fat while they are growing. Without fat, we could not metabolise the fat-soluble vitamins A, D, E and K. Fats also help build cell walls and healthy skin, hair and nails.

Because fats make food taste good, it is very easy to go overboard and eat too much of them. And it's especially bad if you are eating too much of the wrong type of fat.

Which fat?

Saturated fats come from animals and are found in dairy products and eggs as well as in meat. They are also found in coconut oil, palm oil and palm kernel oil. These fats are solid at room temperature – think of butter and the fatty parts of meat. While all fats have the same number of calories, saturated fats are particularly harmful because the body uses them to produce cholesterol, a waxy substance that ends up lining and eventually clogging veins

Oily fish contains Omega-3 polyunsaturated fat, which has been found to reduce the risk of heart disease.

and arteries. Cutting down on saturated fat is an important step in reducing cholesterol levels.

However, other fats, in moderation, can actually help to protect you from heart disease. Oily fish, such as herring, mackerel, salmon, tuna and sardines, have been found to reduce the risk of heart disease. They contain Omega-3 polyunsaturated fat. Corn oil, cotton seed oil, safflower oil, sunflower oil and soy oils are also polyunsaturated. Choosing these oils, whether in liquid form or as margarine, is better for your heart.

Monounsaturated oils are the third group of oils. They are found in olive oil, peanut oil, sesame seeds, canola oil and avocados. These oils are also good for your heart, in moderation.

Hydrogenated fats are highly processed fats which contain trans-fatty acids. These are often found in processed foods since they help preserve food or give it a more appealing texture. They may appear on the label as hydrogenated vegetable oil. Avoid these fats, since they act much like saturated fats within your body.

Working with a healthy diet

A healthy diet doesn't necessarily mean giving up all the foods you love, but it does mean cutting down on fat and sugar, eating more fibre and complex carbohydrates, and probably eating smaller servings of protein-rich foods (a serving of meat should be no more than 80g/ 3 ounces). You can still eat a lot – both in terms of the amount and the types of food. The key is to make your regular food choices healthy by filling your plate with

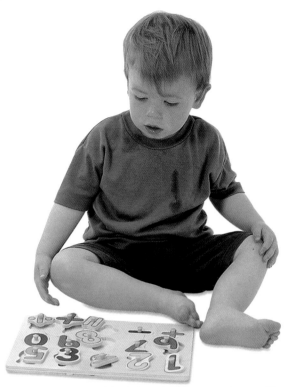

Introducing a healthy, balanced diet at an early age will help avoid problems later on in life.

A word on drinking

Alcohol is full of calories and lacks nutrients. It has been linked to an increased risk of breast cancer in women. Although the recommended limit is 21 units per week for men and 14 for women, it is better for your health to keep well below that. However, red wine plays a part in the famous 'Mediterranean diet', which has been linked to a reduced rate of heart disease so, if you enjoy it, a small glass each day may even be slightly beneficial.

Water is the best drink – natural, calorie-free and cheap. Drinking plenty of water helps your body, particularly if you are exercising hard. To replace the water you lose by exercising, drink two glasses before you start, keep some water handy and sip it while you are exercising, and then drink another couple of glasses when you have finished your workout.

fruit, vegetables and grains, while cutting back on high-fat foods.

Fat has a way of creeping into our diets. Pasta is a healthy choice, but add a rich sauce full of cream and cheese and it becomes a high-fat meal. Salad is great, but salad dressing adds fat. A baked potato has only about 100 calories and almost no fat, but add a tablespoon of butter and you double the calories. Prepared low-fat sauces and dressings are a better choice. Plain lemon juice tastes great on salad and vegetables, while a simple tomato sauce is a healthier choice for pasta.

A healthy diet has room for everything in moderation, so there is no need to give up a particular food altogether. If you love cheese, cut down on it, but don't cut it out. Similarly, eating chocolate or ice cream once in a while is fine.

A baked potato is an excellent low-fat, high-fibre food – but adding butter doubles the calorie content.

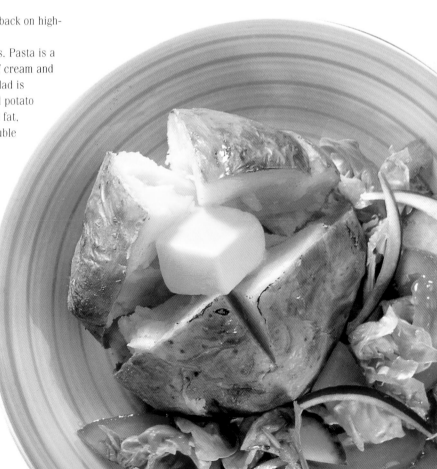

losing *body fat*

Although eating sensibly is the key to maintaining a healthy weight, it may be necessary to diet in order to get down to the right weight. Height and weight charts will tell you if you are the right weight for your height. Remember, however, that muscle weighs more than fat, so if you are muscular your weight may be at the high end for your height.

How to do it sensibly

A sensible diet for weight loss is very similar to any healthy diet, except that fewer calories are consumed. Eating smaller portions and eating less fat will help reduce calories. There is no need, however, to count the calories in every mouthful.

Weight loss should be gradual. Losing more than two pounds per week is not effective in the long run. Quick,

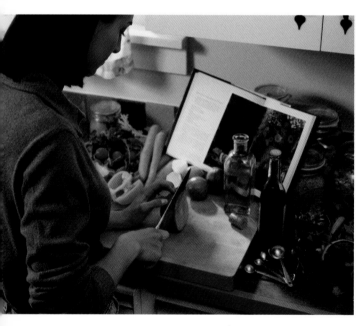

It may take a little longer to prepare fresh foods, but the health benefits make it a very worthwhile exercise.

dramatic weight loss is usually the result of either losing water weight or of following a diet that is dangerously low in calories. Diets that have fewer than 1200 calories per day make your body go into starvation mode, reducing metabolism to conserve weight so that it is actually harder to lose weight. Very restrictive diets are also hard to stick to because they are dull.

Although most people will lose weight on a diet, few dieters manage to keep the weight off. Most people actually gain back the weight once they stop dieting, and even add a few extra pounds. The key to lasting weight loss is changing your eating habits, not just for the duration of the diet, but for the rest of your life. You need to teach yourself new, healthy eating habits and make them part of your life.

In order to teach yourself new habits, you need to educate yourself about foods. In general, fruits and vegetables, when cooked and served without added fat or sugar, can be eaten in large quantities. Changing to low-fat dairy products is another good habit to start. Some cooking methods, such as deep-fat frying, sautéing and shallow frying, add fat to foods, while others such as baking, grilling, steaming, boiling and stir-frying in small amounts of oil add very little. To add flavour, use citrus juices, herbs and spices, not butter, oil and salt.

A simple and healthy diet to follow is based on the recommended daily amount of the various food groups: six servings of carbohydrates, two servings of fruit, two servings of vegetables, two servings of low-fat dairy products and two servings of protein. Remember that the serving size is small. A serving of protein is about 80 g (3 oz), while a serving of carbohydrate is half a cup of cooked pasta or one slice of bread. These are almost certainly much smaller servings than you are used to. To help fill you up and get more vitamins, take extra servings of tomatoes, vegetables from the cabbage family (cabbage, broccoli, cauliflower) and salad vegetables (celery, cucumber, lettuce, radishes, carrots).

Use butter and oil sparingly, only one tablespoon per day in total. If you can't resist the occasional biscuit or sweet, cut out one of your carbohydrate servings, or cut down on fat.

For support and inspiration, try joining a slimming club or buying a book of low-fat recipes. When selecting a weight-loss programme or book, do not choose one that promises rapid weight loss of more than 900 g (2lb) per week, or that promises to take weight off some areas of your body rather than others. Spot weight reduction is not possible, while rapid weight loss is not healthy. Methods that focus on gradual weight loss, healthy eating habits and realistic targets are healthier and work better in the long run.

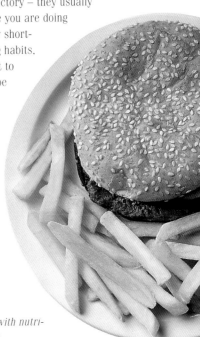

No more crash diets

Crash diets are very unsatisfactory – they usually make you feel miserable while you are doing them, and the effects are very short-lived. By changing your eating habits, you will no longer need to diet to lose weight. Instead you will be able to enjoy eating a variety of foods because you will know which foods to choose.

Exercising at the same time will help you lose weight faster, as well as toning your muscles. Since exercising burns up calories, and losing weight is the process of taking in fewer calories than you burn, burning extra calories through exercise makes sense.

Fresh whole foods are packed with nutrients, unlike fat-laden fast food!

Keep an eye on your waist measurement to monitor whether you are gaining weight.

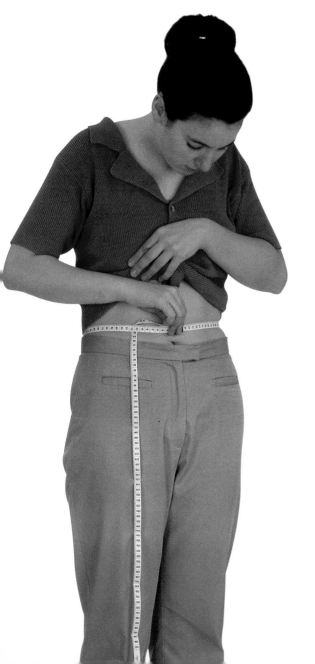

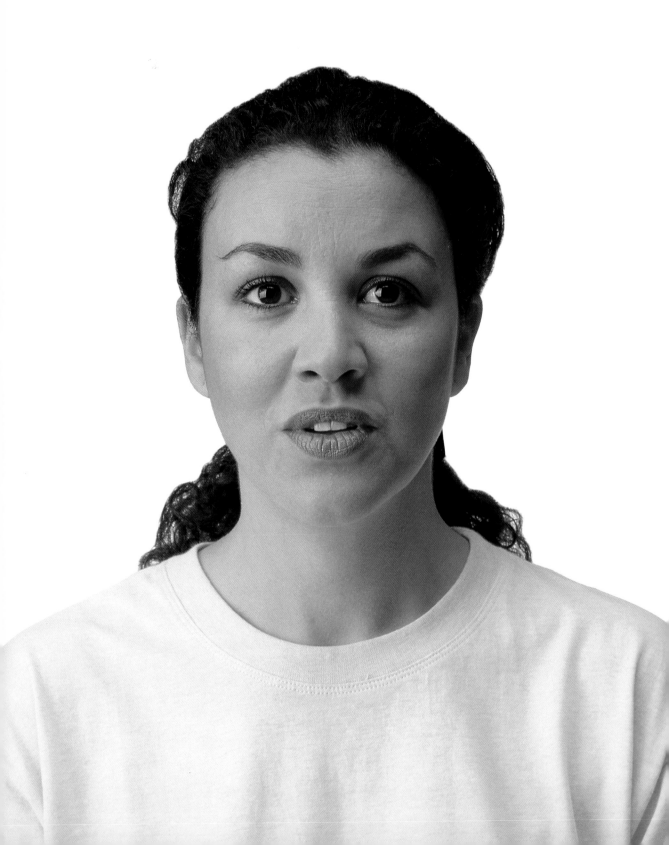

6   MotivatingYourself

Half the battle with exercise is about getting motivated to start, and then keeping it up on a regular basis – but there are plenty of good reasons for making the effort. When you exercise regularly, you will notice not only a physical change in your shape but also an increasing feeling of mental and emotional well-being. After a while, you will probably find that you are sleeping better, feeling more in control and less stressed. A few simple, practical steps can help you get motivated to start exercising and keep exercising. You will need to be patient with yourself at first. Exercise is a habit that you are trying to develop – breaking a bad habit doesn't happen quickly, and starting a good habit takes time too. The important thing is to get yourself into the right frame of mind, with the help of positive visualisations and affirmations if necessary.

exercising *your mind*

Regular exercise can make you feel mentally and emotionally better – but have you thought about using your mind and your emotions to help yourself before you exercise? With a bit of positive thinking, you can motivate yourself to start an exercise programme, keep yourself on track, or work out more effectively. The way to do this is to change your attitude towards yourself.

The feel-good factor

During exercise, hormones are released in the brain. These hormones – called endorphins – are both calming and mood elevating. Quite simply, they make people feel good. When people who exercise regularly say that it is addictive, they often mean that they are addicted to the wonderful feeling of well-being they get when they have completed their workout.

Motivating yourself

Before you embark on your exercise programme, get yourself organised with both a practical and a mental plan of attack.

Regular sessions will help you get into the exercise habit. You need to set aside time for exercise, whether it's daily or three times a week. Make an appointment with yourself. Write it down in your diary, then set an alarm to remind yourself. And don't break your date. If circumstances mean you have to miss a session, don't give up – just make sure to keep your exercise date next time. Make sure also that you have any equipment and clothes ready, so that you are not tempted to skip a session for want of a clean pair of leggings!

Getting fit won't happen overnight. It's a gradual process. If you have unrealistic expectations, you are setting yourself up for failure, and feeling that you have failed is a sure-fire demotivator. Instead, set realistic, achievable goals. The aim is to stretch yourself without getting discouraged.

Negative versus positive language

Just as the action of hormones in your body has an effect on your brain, so your brain can have some strong effects on your body. Telling yourself that you are doing well can make you do even better, while telling yourself that you are doing badly sets you up for certain failure.

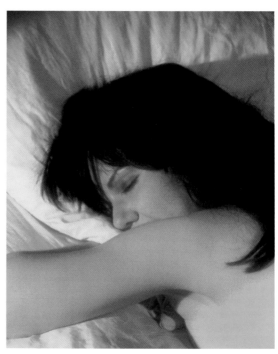

Before you fall asleep at night, give yourself a mental pat on the back for the good things you've achieved that day.

To see how true this is, recall a time when you were doing something physical, such as playing tennis or bouncing a ball, effortlessly. If you suddenly think 'I'm not going to be able to keep this up!', you will almost certainly fumble the ball.

Everyone talks to themselves, but have you ever listened to how you talk to yourself? Think about it for a moment. Do you focus on things you've done wrong? ('I nearly had an accident. Typical!') Do you call yourself names, such as 'Clumsy' or 'Idiot'? Do you belittle yourself ('I'm a terrible driver')? This is called negative self-talk and it is hazardous to your health.

When we talk to ourselves like this, we are sending negative messages to the unconscious. We are reinforcing the bad feelings we have about ourselves. Think back to when you were in school. Do you remember how badly you did in classes where the teacher expected the worst of you? That teacher sent out negative messages, making it almost impossible for you to learn or do well.

Now think of someone who gave out positive messages, believing that you could do something and telling you so. You almost certainly did better when you were around that person. They gave you confidence, which made everything easier.

Positive self-talk is a way to give yourself confidence by making the voice inside your head help you to do and be your best. If you are talking positively to yourself you might say, 'I look really nice in this dress', or 'I did a good job at work today', or 'I'm a good and loving friend'.

Listen to what the little voice inside you is saying. If you are already saying good things to yourself and patting yourself on the back, well done! If your internal voice is critical or negative, don't worry. Just start introducing some positive words. It might feel silly at first. You might even feel that you shouldn't give yourself compliments. Many people have been taught from childhood not to

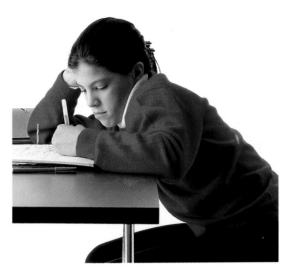

Negative feedback is uninspiring. Children may not learn well in classes where a teacher has a low opinion of them.

brag or call attention to their good points. Don't worry if you have those feelings – just give positive self-talk a go for a week or two. It will start to feel more natural after a while.

Think yourself fit

You can use positive self-talk while you are exercising to improve your workout. Tell yourself you are doing a good job. Always focus on what you are getting right, not on what you are doing wrong. If you spot yourself doing a movement awkwardly, congratulate yourself for noticing your mistake and don't beat yourself up for not being perfect.

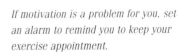

If motivation is a problem for you, set an alarm to remind you to keep your exercise appointment.

using your *sense organs*

Most people respond more positively to one of their senses than to the others – some are visual, others respond to sounds. A third group is more receptive to feelings and movement. Once you have identified which is your dominant sense, you can use your natural bent to make exercise more effective and more fun – and learn how to activate your less dominant senses, too.

Which is your dominant sense?

People with a strong visual sense tend to say things like 'I see what you mean'. Those with an auditory bent are more likely to say 'I like the sound of that'. People who approach the world through feelings and movement – kinaesthetically – use expressions like 'I have a good feeling about that'.

Similarly, if someone asks you a neutral question such as 'What was your holiday like?' and you look straight ahead as you answer, you are picturing what it looked like; if you look down and left you are remembering the sounds, and if you look down and right you are recalling how it felt to be there. (Left-handed people sometimes do the opposite, however.)

Visual people are motivated by appearances and colour, and prefer to read instructions rather than listen to them. People with a strong auditory sense love music and can use it to motivate themselves. They take in more through the spoken word. People who grasp the world through their kinaesthetic senses enjoy being active and learn best by doing.

How to develop your senses

If you are a visual person, try listening to music more or bring in your kinaesthetic sense by taking a walk as you look at the view. If you love being active, try exercising to music or developing your visual sense by drawing with brightly coloured crayons. If your auditory sense is strongest, try moving to the music to stimulate your

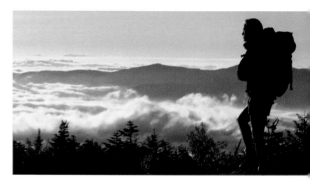

Visual people are inspired by beautiful scenery.

kinaesthetic sense or watching television with the sound off to expand your visual perception.

Using your senses to get more out of exercise

Visual people are motivated by looks, so an attractive exercise outfit is a good investment. Sports with a beautiful image, such as ballet or riding, or those that allow visual people to enjoy the scenery, such as cycling, walking or running, may appeal.

Auditory people are motivated by sound and music and will probably work well to audio tapes. Dance and exercising to music attract people whose auditory sense is well developed.

Kinaesthetic people enjoy exercise because it makes them feel good. Ball games that involve movement as well as hand-eye co-ordination are fun for them. They may also enjoy the total body experience of swimming.

a positive mind

A positive mental attitude sets the stage for success because it does not allow thoughts of failure. If you really believe that something is possible, you are more likely to make it happen. If you tend to have negative expectations, and they are usually fulfilled (whether you wanted them to be or not!), then it follows that positive expectations can also be fulfilled – if you allow yourself to have them.

Using affirmations

One way to become more positive is by repeating an affirmation – a positive statement that will help develop beliefs that are good for you, such as 'I love my exercise routine' or 'I am fit and healthy'.

Thoughts like 'I hate doing my exercises, but it's the only way to get the body I want' are demotivating and make you dread exercise, so replace those negative messages with affirmations. Decide what you would like to believe about exercise, then write your wishes down as a series of positive statements, such as 'Exercise is fun', or 'I love it when I work my hardest'. Repeat your affirmations firmly – either to yourself or out loud – five or six times in a row, two or three times a day. Alternatively, you can write them down and stick them where you will see them often – on the fridge or a mirror. Pretty soon you will start to believe them.

Bring your positive affirmations to mind as you start your exercise session.

Using your feelings to assess how hard you work

Listen to your body to assess how hard you are working. When you exercise aerobically, you should be working out at a pace that leaves you out of breath but still able to carry on a conversation. If you can't talk, slow down until you can say a few words. If you aren't out of breath at all, speed up – you're not working hard enough! Think of a scale marked with numbers from one to ten, with one being at rest and ten exercising your hardest. You should be exercising at level six or seven.

Giving your all

When you start an exercise session, bring your affirmations to mind and get out your mental scale to measure how hard you are working. Now put your three senses – visual, auditory and kinaesthetic – into gear. Use your visual sense to create an image of how you should look during exercise and how you want your body to be – toned and fit. Add your auditory sense by telling yourself what you're going to do and repeating your affirmations to yourself. Then bring in the kinaesthetic sense by thinking about how your muscles are going to feel during the exercises. You can also ask your muscles to work harder.

visualisations

A visualisation is a private movie that you run in your mind's eye. You can use visualisation to change your attitudes and behaviours, to create positive feelings and to help achieve your goals. Therapists use visualisations to help people recover from illness. A cancer patient might be asked to visualise chemotherapy drugs or white blood cells killing off the cancer cells.

Why visualise?

Athletes use visualisation to improve performance. A figure skater, for example, might go over her routine in her mind, seeing it happening perfectly time after time. This process is also called mental rehearsal.

Many people use visualisations for relaxation. They might sit or lie quietly and recall in great detail a time when they were perfectly relaxed and at ease. They would hear the waves lapping on the shore and the birds singing in the trees, enjoy the warm sun on their shoulders, feel the deck-chair cradling them comfortably, see the blue of the sea and the white sand.

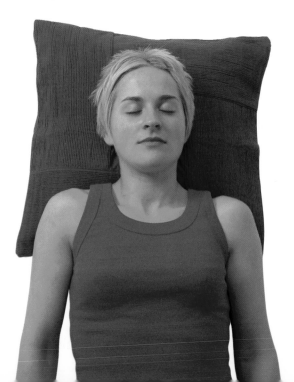

Relaxation

The first step to visualisation is relaxation. First, prepare a peaceful environment – take the phone off the hook and shut the door. Your might like to vaporise your favourite relaxing aromatherapy oil, or play some soothing music very quietly. Now sit or lie down comfortably. One of the simplest ways to relax is a technique called progressive muscular relaxation. Start with your head and scrunch up your face, then loosen and relax it. Work your way down your whole body from head to toes, tightening then relaxing each muscle group. When you have finished, your whole body will be relaxed.

Now take a moment to think about your breathing. Take deep, slow, comfortable breaths. Breathe in through your nose and out through your mouth. As you breathe, your stomach will expand. Let it expand as far as it will go naturally, without forcing it. Take air deep into your lungs, letting them fill up, rather than just breathing from the top of your chest.

Visualisation

Now that you are fully relaxed, you can create your visualisation. To improve your body image, imagine someone stroking your body lovingly and telling you that you are beautiful. Let them linger on the parts of your body that you don't love. Look into the future and see

Learn a relaxation technique, such as progressive muscular relaxation, to help prepare you for a visualisation session.

your body changing step by step, your tummy getting firmer, your bottom toned. Or, you might want to see yourself radiating health and feeling happy. If you want to improve your diet, you could visualise yourself enjoying delicious fresh fruits and vegetables, knowing when you feel full and stopping just then.

You can improve your exercise technique by imagining yourself doing your exercise routine perfectly. Make the picture really detailed. Listen to the sounds of your breathing, feel your muscles working. Focus on your muscles and encourage them to work harder. If you want to work on your posture, visualise yourself standing perfectly straight and tall, your back in a nice line, your bottom tucked in and your tummy pulled up, your head nicely balanced. Think of how this will feel in your muscles and of how you will look.

Sample visualisation

It's hard to relax while you are reading instructions from a book, so get a tape recorder and read the following section, slowly and clearly, pausing after each sentence. Then lie down comfortably, spend some time relaxing your muscles and breathing deeply, and when you are ready, hit the play button.

'Relax even more deeply (pause) and slow down your breathing even more (pause). You are now fully relaxed and breathing deeply and slowly. Today you are going to watch yourself become stronger and fitter. Close your eyes.

'You are standing in your exercise outfit. Your music comes on. You tap your foot and sway a little, enjoying the sound. You start your workout. You feel really good and moving makes you feel even better. As you march on the spot to warm up, you can see yourself standing straight and tall. You look comfortable and relaxed. You feel happy. As you get into your routine, you realise that you are having fun. You smile. Your muscles

are working well and effortlessly. You feel warm and loose. Your shoulders and hands are relaxed, your tummy is firm and pulled in, your bottom is tight and toned. You see yourself and your body as you are in the future. You love the way you look. Freeze frame – see yourself looking and feeling good. Let yourself really feel and see the new you. Take a deep breath. Open your eyes.'

You can create visualisations to suit yourself. Writing them down, and then reciting them into a tape recorder so that you can listen to them during your relaxation sessions, is a good way to help you achieve your goals.

Visualise yourself radiating health and feeling happy – and soon you will be!

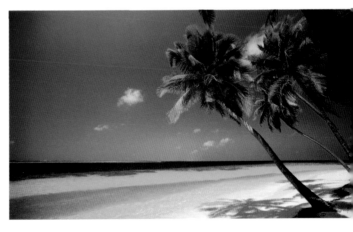

Unwind by visualising somewhere you have felt relaxed – perhaps your favourite holiday beach.

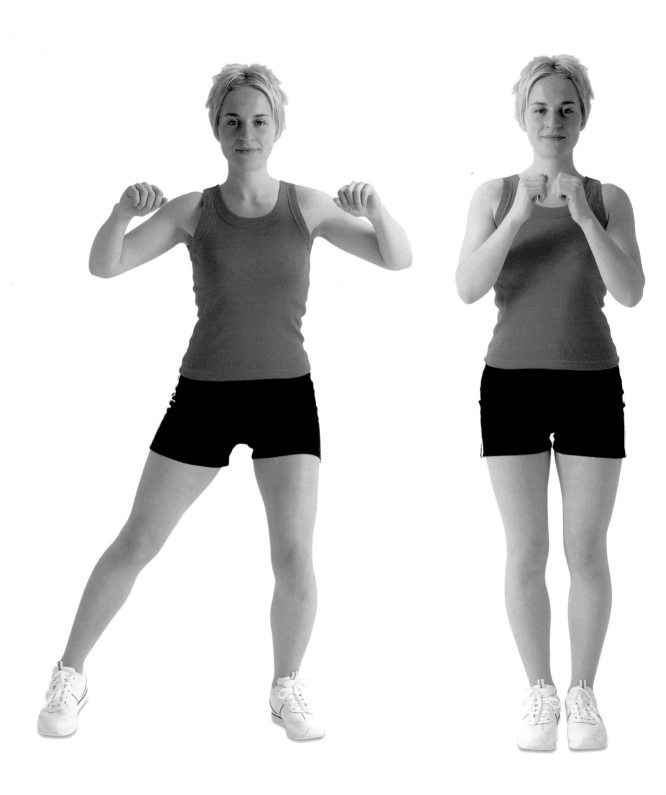

7 WarmingUp

The initial warm-up is an essential part of any exercise programme,
and you must make sure that you allow enough time to include it.
Not only does the warm-up prepare you for the work about to be
done by gently engaging the muscles you will be using, it also
reduces the risk of injury by stimulating the circulation and literally warming you up. When the body is cold, the muscles and
joints are less pliable and are therefore more prone to being
strained. The warm-up also gets you ready mentally for the
exercise you are about to do, giving you a few minutes to release
any mental or physical tension you are holding in the body before
you start the workout. This is time you have set aside for your
own benefit, so start focusing all your attention on yourself and
concentrate on your technique.

doing it *correctly*

By now you will have assessed your fitness level, started making any necessary changes to your diet, and talked yourself into a positive state of mind! Affirmations and visualisations will be part of your daily routine, and you are now ready to start taking action towards that sleek new you. Take a few moments to remind yourself of the five golden rules below, and you're ready to start warming up.

Breathe easy

Breathing is something we all do without thinking, but when it comes to exercise, it's important to concentrate on breathing correctly and effectively. A common mistake is to hold the breath, which restricts the amount of oxygen entering the body and can also raise the blood pressure.

Take *five*

1   *It's a good idea to plan when you are going to exercise. Mark it in your diary, choosing a time that will suit you best on most days – and stick to it! Your body will soon become programmed to working out at this time.*

2   *Remember to start gradually and build up your exercise programme. It takes time to get fit and toned.*

3   *Wear loose comfortable clothing, so your skin can breathe and sweat is carried from the surface of the skin.*

4   *Check your footwear – trainers or a pair of supportive walking shoes are a must.*

5   *Always check with your GP before starting any new exercise programme.*

1   Sit on the floor with your legs crossed, keeping your back straight and your chest lifted.

2   Lower your head and close your eyes. Now concentrate on your breathing.

3   Place your hands on your stomach, fingertips either side of your navel. Inhale slowly through your nose, making sure the air fills your stomach and pushes out your navel.

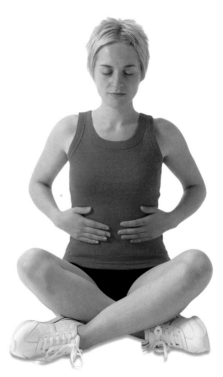

4 Exhale through your mouth, making a forceful blowing sound as you do so.

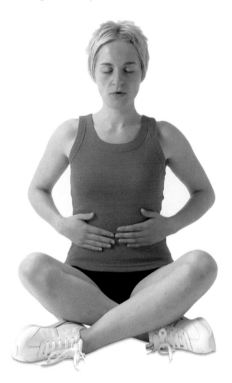

5 Tighten your abs at the end of the breath out.

When exercising, the general rule is to breathe out with each effort, which means you breathe in just before a movement takes place, and exhale during the effort of the movement. This ensures that your abs are engaged and avoids a 'domed' effect developing in the tummy – which is the opposite of what you are aiming for.

The warm-up

With the following exercise programme, you will be working the bum and tum areas and therefore you need to loosen the spine, the pelvis and the hip joints in the warm-up. If you decide to work only one area on a particular day, then just perform the appropriate warm-up exercises for that muscle group.

Warm-up exercises for the bum

- Pelvic tilt
- Hip circles
- Knee bends
- Toe taps, side and behind

Warm-up exercises for the tum

- Pelvic tilt
- Waist twists
- Spinal curl
- Side bends

Marching on the spot after you have performed these moves will help to raise your body temperature. Once you feel warm and loose, spend a few minutes stretching out the muscles. Hold each stretch position for about 10–15 seconds. When you come to cool down at the end of the programme, stretches should be held for up to 30 seconds. This will help lengthen the muscles that have been worked and reduce stiffness.

bum

exercises...*warm-up*

 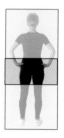

10 MINS

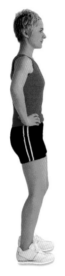 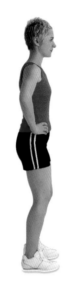

Pelvic tilt

1 Stand with your feet hip-width apart, knees slightly bent, your upper body relaxed.
2 Tighten your abs.
3 Gently tilt your pelvis forward, then return to the neutral position.
4 Gently tilt the pelvis backward, then return to the neutral position.
5 Repeat five times, front and back.

Remember ...
• *Your posture – stand tall.*
• *Abs are held in tight.*

NOTE: You can practise this movement throughout the day, not just when you're exercising.

 KEEP ALL MOVEMENTS SLOW AND CONTROLLED

Hip circles

1 Stand with your feet hip-width apart, knees slightly bent and your upper body relaxed.
2 Tighten your abs.
3 Gently rock your pelvis backward and forward, then side to side, until the movement becomes a circle.
4 Do 8–12 circles to the right, then 8–12 to the left.

Remember ...
• *Your posture – your body is centred as you circle the hips.*

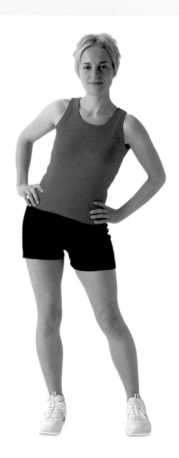

Knee bends

1 Stand with your feet hip-width apart, hands on your hips, feet slightly turned out.
2 Tighten your abs.
3 Keep your upper body relaxed.

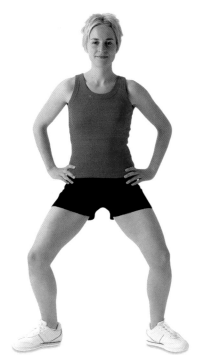

4 Gently bend your knees, then straighten, keeping your knees slightly bent when you come up.
5 Do one set (8–12 repetitions).

Remember …
• *Don't lock your knees.*
• *Keep your knees in line with your toes – don't go beyond them.*
• *Keep your bottom tucked under.*

Marching

1 To raise your body temperature, march on the spot, pumping your arms backward and forward, for 1 minute.
2 Start low and gradually raise your knees higher.

Toe taps to the back

1 Stand with your feet hip-width apart, hands on your hips.
2 Leaning slightly forward, tap your right foot to the back, then bring back to the centre.
3 Change legs.
4 Keep a steady rhythm with the movement and continue toe tapping to the back until your body starts to feel warm.

Remember …
• *The back heel remains off the ground.*
• *Squeeze your bottom.*
• *Abs are held in tight.*

NOTE: You can bring both your arms forward, to shoulder height, as you toe tap to the back.

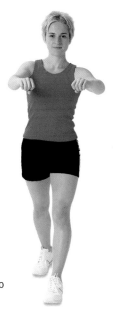

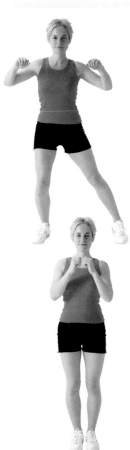

Toe taps to the side

1 Stand with your feet hip-width apart, your hands on your hips.
2 Tap your left leg to the side, raising both arms out to the side as you do so, then bring back to the centre.
3 Change legs.
4 Keep a steady rhythm to the movement and continue toe tapping to the side until your body starts to feel warm.

Remember …
• *Knees remain slightly bent throughout.*
• *Arms go to shoulder-height only.*
• *Abs are held in tight.*

tum
exercises...*warm-up*

 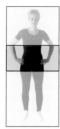

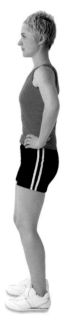 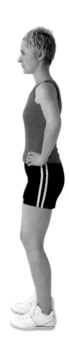 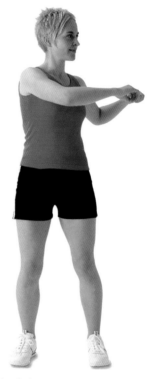

Pelvic tilt

1 Stand with your feet hip-width apart, knees slightly bent, upper body relaxed.

2 Tighten your abs.

3 Gently tilt your pelvis forward, then return to the neutral position.

4 Gently tilt the pelvis backward, then return to the neutral position.

5 Repeat five times, front and back.

Remember ...
- *Your posture – stand tall.*
- *Abs are held in tight.*

NOTE: You can practise this movement throughout the day, not just when you're exercising.

Waist twists

1 Stand with your feet hip-width apart, knees slightly bent, your spine in a neutral position.

2 Tighten your abs.

3 Clasp your hands loosely in front of you, at shoulder height.

4 Keeping your hips still and facing forward, gently twist your shoulders and head around to one side, then return to centre.

5 Twist your shoulders and head around to the other side, then return to centre.

6 Repeat five times, right and left.

Remember ...
- *Your posture: chest high, abs in, back straight.*
- *Hips and knees face forward.*

Side bends

1 Stand with your feet hip-width apart, knees slightly bent, your spine in a neutral position.
2 Tighten your abs.
3 Gently slide one hand down the side of your leg to feel a stretch in the waist.
4 Slowly return to centre and repeat on the other side.
5 Repeat five times each side.

Remember ...
- *Don't lean forward.*
- *Bend only as far as is comfortable.*
- *Keep your shoulders back and over your hips.*

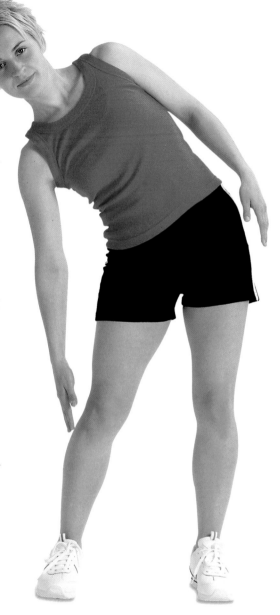

Spinal curl

1 Stand with your feet shoulder-width apart, knees slightly bent and your body leaning slightly forward.
2 Rest your hands on your thighs for support.
3 Your back should be flat and your abs tight.
4 Gently lift up through the spine and round your back.
5 Hold, then release down to the neutral, flat-back position.

Remember ...
- *Your posture – chest high, abs in, back straight.*
- *Hips and knees face forward.*
- *Keep your shoulders relaxed.*
- *Don't over-arch your back.*

NOTE: This exercise can also be done on the floor. Kneel down on all fours, with your hands directly under your shoulders and your knees directly under your hips. Your back should be flat and your abs tight. Gently lift up through the spine and round your back. Hold, then release down to the neutral, flat-back position.

Marching

1 To raise your body temperature, march on the spot, pumping your arms backward and forward, for 1 minute.
2 Start low and gradually raise your knees higher.

> ! KEEP ALL MOVEMENTS SLOW AND CONTROLLED

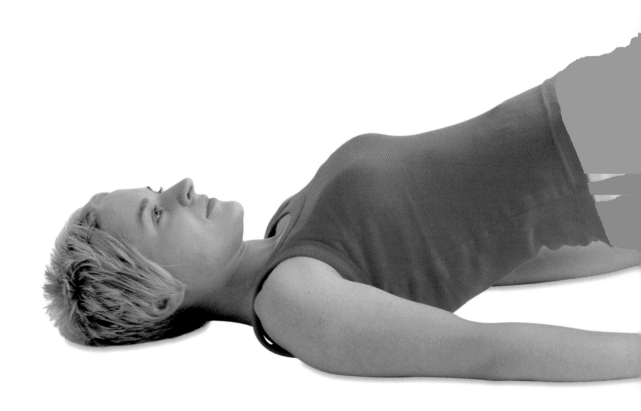

8   Beginner's Workout

You are now warmed up and ready to start on the beginner's

workout. The most important thing to bear in mind when doing

the exercises is to keep all movements slow and controlled – it's

the quality of the movements that counts, not the quantity, so

focus on perfecting your technique. Remember to keep your back

flat and your abs pulled in tightly at all times, and make sure you

are working the correct muscles – if you lose concentration or

start to tire, it is all too easy to let a stronger group of muscles

kick in and take over. Work through the whole routine at your

own pace – it is better to complete all the exercises comfortably

at first by doing just a few repetitions than to run out of energy

half-way through. You can aim to increase the number of

repetitions each time you do the workout.

bum
exercises...*beginner's*

 10 MINS

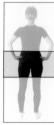

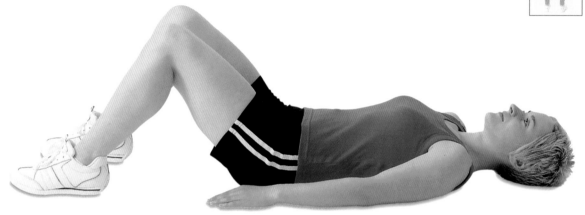

Buttock squeeze

1 Lie on your back, knees bent, with your hands by your sides.

2 Tighten your abs and tilt your pelvis as you would in a pelvic tilt.

3 Keeping your abs tight, gently lift your hips off the floor and squeeze your bottom, then release.

4 Build up to 20 repetitions.

Remember …
• *Keep your hips still.*

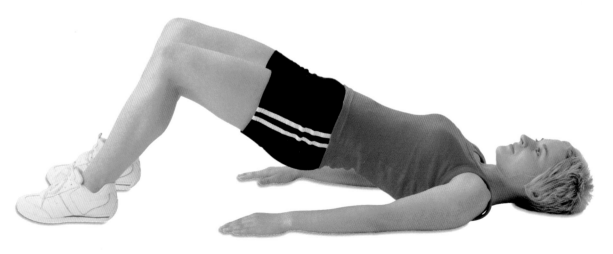

Squats

1 Stand with your feet shoulder-width apart, toes facing forward.

2 Place your hands on your hips.

3 Bend your knees as if you're about to sit down in a chair, sticking your bottom out to the back.

4 Push through the heels to come up to a standing position, keeping your knees slightly bent as you do so.

5 Do one set (8–12 repetitions).

Remember …
- *Your back remains flat throughout.*
- *Don't lock your knees.*

NOTE: You can have your arms crossed over your chest or extending forward, to shoulder height, as you squat down.

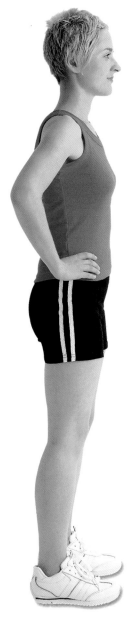
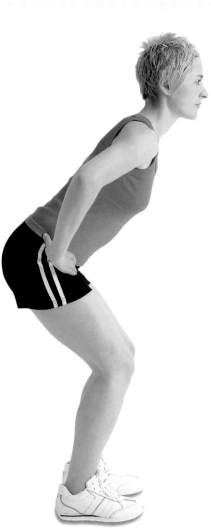

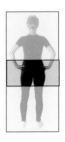

Outer thigh raise

1 Lie on one side, hips facing forward, thighs together and your body in a straight line.
2 Support your head in one hand and place the other hand on the floor in front of you for support.

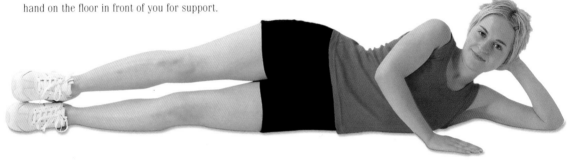

3 Bend both knees back.

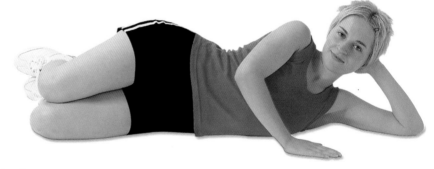

4 Gently raise the top leg, then lower.
5 Do one set (6–7 repetitions), then repeat on the other side.

Remember …
• Squeeze your buttocks as you raise and lower your leg.
• Hips face forward.

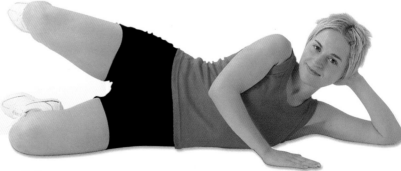

Inner thigh raise

1 Lie on your side, hips facing forward, thighs together and your body in a straight line.

2 Support your head in one hand and place the other hand on the floor in front of you for support.

3 Bend your top leg over in front of you, resting your knee on a cushion if you like.

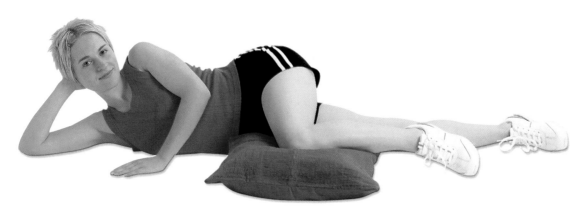

4 Lift the underneath extended leg, keeping the knee slightly bent, then lower.

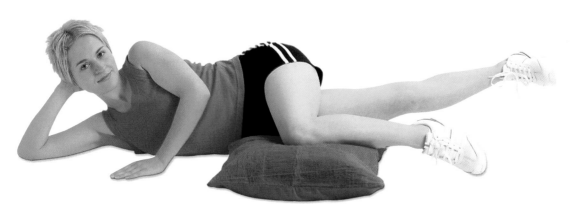

5 Do one set (8–12 repetitions), then repeat on the other side.

Remember …
- *Foot and hips face forward.*
- *Keep both knees slightly bent.*

bum
stretches...*beginner's*

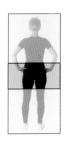 10 MINS

Hip flexor stretch

1 Stand tall with your feet hip-width apart.

2 Step back with the right leg, bend both knees and lift the right heel off the floor.

3 Keep your pelvis tucked under, and hold. Repeat on the other leg.

Remember ...
- *Your posture – upper body is upright.*
- *Hips and feet face forward.*
- *Abs are held in tight.*

Quad/front of thigh stretch

1 Stand tall with your feet hip-width apart, knees slightly bent.

2 Lift and bend one leg up behind you and hold the ankle with your hand.

3 Keep your knees aligned and the knee of the bent leg facing the floor, hips pushing slightly forward.

4 Hold, then repeat on the other leg.

5 Feel the stretch at the front of the thigh.

Remember ...
- *Your posture – upper body is upright.*
- *Abs are held in tight.*

NOTE: You can use a wall or chair for support if you can't keep your balance in this position.

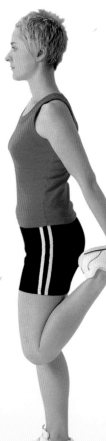

Buttock stretch

1 Stand tall with your feet hip-width apart, knees slightly bent.

2 Bring the ankle of one leg up and across the knee of the supporting leg, so that it looks as if you're crossing your legs standing up.

3 Keeping your ankle over your knee, pull your abs in tight and bend your supporting leg.

4 Hold, then repeat on the other leg.

Remember …
- *Your upper body can lean forward slightly.*
- *Hips stay centred; back remains flat.*
- *Keep your head in line with your body.*

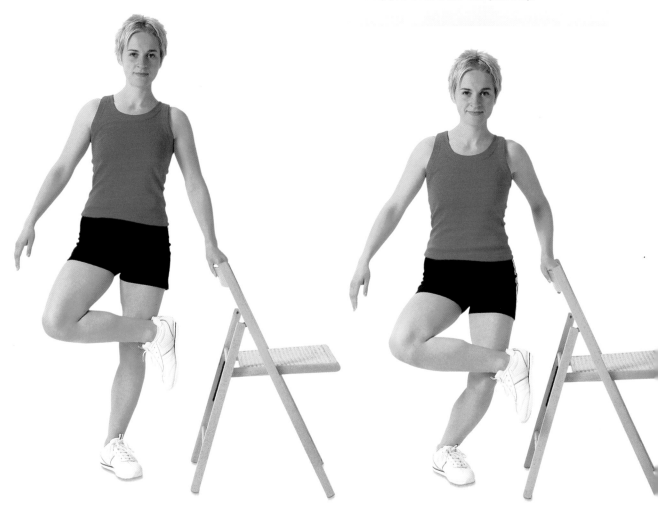

HOLD THESE STRETCHES FOR 6–10 SECONDS IN THE WARM-UP, GRADUALLY BUILDING UP TO 30 SECONDS IN THE COOL-DOWN

Inner thigh stretch

1 Stand tall with your feet wider than shoulder-width apart and turned out slightly.
2 Bend one leg to the side, keeping the other leg straight, with the foot on the floor.
3 Place your hands on your thighs for support and lean forward slightly.
4 Hold, then repeat on the other side.

Remember …
• *Your posture – upper body is lifted.*
• *Knees are in line with your toes.*

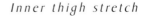

Hamstring stretch

1 Stand tall with your feet hip-width apart.
2 Extend one leg forward and bend the other slightly.
3 Pull up from the spine and pull in your abs as you gently lean forward from the hips; pressing your hips further behind will increase the stretch.
4 Lift your tail bone to the ceiling and feel the stretch in the back of the thigh.
5 Hold, then repeat on the other side.

Remember …
• *Your posture – chest is lifted, back is straight, head is looking forward.*

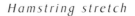

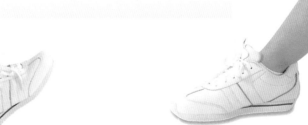

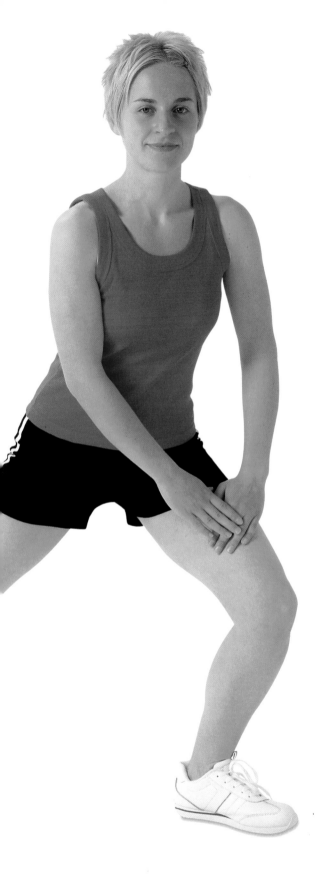

bum programme

Spend about 30 seconds on each exercise on each side (when worked separately).

Warm-up

1 Pelvic tilt
2 Hip circles
3 Knee bends
4 Toe taps, side and behind
5 Marching on the spot until you feel warm
6 Stretch
Hold each stretch for 6–10 seconds:
• Quad stretch
• Hamstring stretch

Toning exercises

1 Buttock squeeze
2 Squats
3 Outer thigh raise
4 Inner thigh raise
5 Stretch
Hold each stretch for 15–30 seconds:
• Hip flexor stretch
• Quad stretch
• Buttock stretch
• Hamstring stretch
• Inner thigh stretch

tum
exercises...*beginner's*

 10 MINS

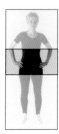

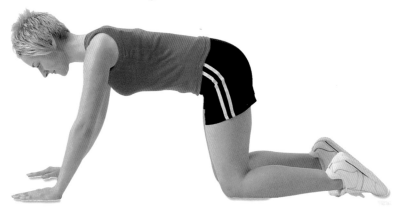

Tummy tightener

1 Kneel down on all fours, with your hands directly under your shoulders, your elbows slightly bent, your knees directly under your hips.
2 Look down at the floor, keeping your head in line with the rest of the body.
3 Relax your abs completely, then slowly pull them up and in tight.
4 Hold for 30 seconds, building up to 1 minute, then relax.

Remember ...
• *Keep your spine still and flat.*
• *Don't lock your elbows.*

Lying pelvic tilts

1 Lie on the floor with your feet hip-width apart, your knees bent.
2 Tighten your abs, keeping your upper body relaxed and your hands by your side.

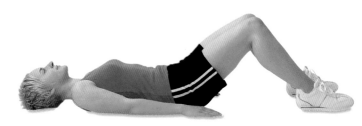

3 Gently squeeze your buttock muscles and tilt your pelvis up, then back down.
4 Repeat the movement, stopping at the half-way point and keeping your spine in a neutral position.
5 Pull your abs in, hold for a count of four, then release for four.
6 Build up to one set (8–12 repetitions).

Remember ...
• *Breathe.*

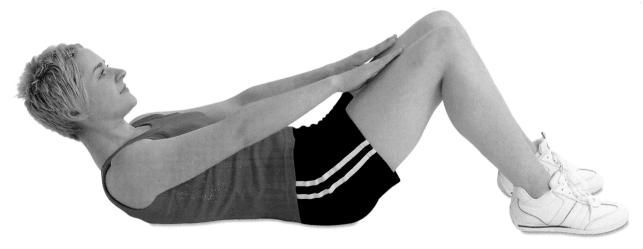

Basic curl-up

1 Lie on the floor with your feet hip-width apart and firmly on the floor, your knees bent.

2 Rest your hands on your thighs.

3 Tilt your pelvis to a neutral position and tighten your abs.

4 Using your tummy muscles, gently lift your shoulders off the floor, then lower.

5 Do one set (8–12 repetitions).

Remember …
• Breathe out when you come up, breathe in when you lower.
• Relax your head and neck and keep your chin off your chest.
• The movement should be fluid and continuous.
• Your back remains on the floor at all times.

Waist tightener/ oblique curls

1 Lie on the floor with your feet hip-width apart and firmly on the floor, with your knees bent.

2 Place your left hand behind your head, with your elbow bent. Place your right foot on your left knee.

3 Place your other hand on the floor for support.

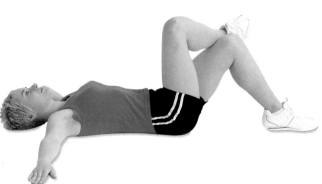

4 Tighten your abs and slowly curl up and over diagonally, bringing your shoulder round to meet your knee, then lower.

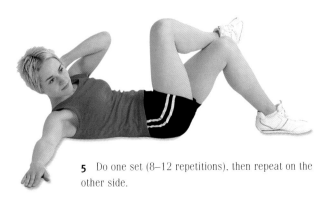

5 Do one set (8–12 repetitions), then repeat on the other side.

tum
stretches...*beginner's*

Abdominal stretch

1 Lie on your stomach, and place your
hands on the floor in front of you at
shoulder level, so that your elbows are
in line with your shoulders.

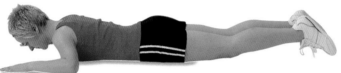

2 Gently push up onto your elbows
by lifting your head and shoulders off
the floor.

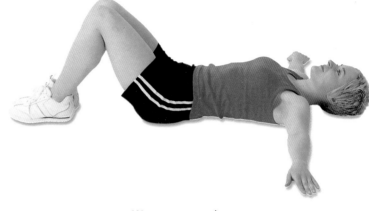

Remember ...
• *Look forward when you lift your
head.*
• *Keep your hips, elbows and feet on
the floor.*

Waist stretch

1 Lie on your back with your knees bent
and your arms at shoulder level.
2 Gently drop both knees to one side and
turn your head in the opposite direction.
3 Hold, then slowly repeat on the
other side.

Remember ...
• *Keep your feet and both shoulders on
the floor.*
• *Breathe easily throughout.*

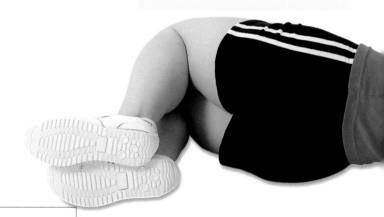

HOLD THESE STRETCHES FOR **6–10** SECONDS IN
THE WARM-UP, GRADUALLY BUILDING UP TO **30**
SECONDS IN THE COOL-DOWN

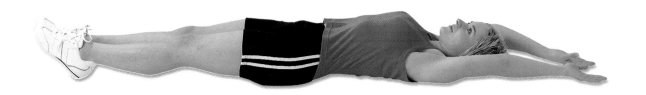

Full body stretch

1 Lie on your back with your arms extended above your head.

2 Gently stretch and lengthen your body, right through your fingertips and down to your toes.

3 Hold for a minimum of 10 seconds, gradually building up to 30 seconds, then gently release and slowly bring your arms down by your side.

Remember ...
- *Breathe gently.*
- *Don't over-arch your back.*

NOTE: Your lower back may come gently off the floor.

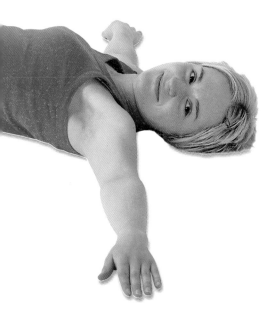

tum programme

Spend about 30 seconds on each exercise on each side (when worked separately).

Warm-up

1 Pelvic tilt
2 Waist twists
3 Side bends
4 Spinal curl
5 Marching on the spot until you feel warm
6 Stretch
Hold the stretch for 6–10 seconds:
- Full body stretch

Toning exercises

1 Tummy tightener
2 Lying pelvic tilt
3 Basic curl-up
4 Waist tightener/oblique curls
5 Stretch
Hold each stretch for 15–30 seconds:
- Ab stretch
- Waist stretch
- Full body stretch

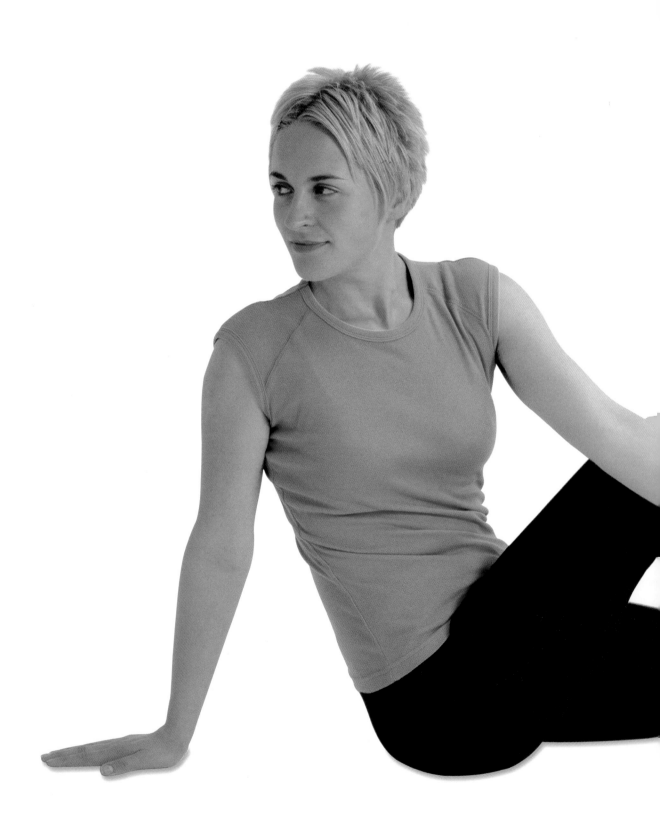

9 IntermediateWorkout

Now that you are becoming familiar with the exercises in the workout, you can really start to concentrate on working the buttock muscles through their full range of movement. As before, keep all the movements slow and controlled, remember to keep breathing easily and naturally, and don't be too ambitious – you can gradually increase the number of sets you do for each exercise as you become stronger. The tummy exercises in this section are also slightly more challenging than the previous ones, but the same rules apply. Work through the routine at your own pace, making sure you concentrate on carrying out the movements properly, using the correct muscles – quality is still more important than quantity. Again, you can gradually increase the time you spend on each exercise or add to the number of repetitions you do as you become stronger.

bum
exercises...*intermediate*

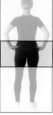

10 MINS

Wide squat

1 Stand tall with your feet a little wider than shoulder-width apart, toes turned out slightly.

2 Your upper body is upright and relaxed, abs and buttock muscles are tight.

3 Place your hands on your hips.

4 Gently bend your knees in line with your toes, then slowly come up.

5 Do one set (8–12 repetitions).

Remember ...
• *Don't lock your knees when you come up.*

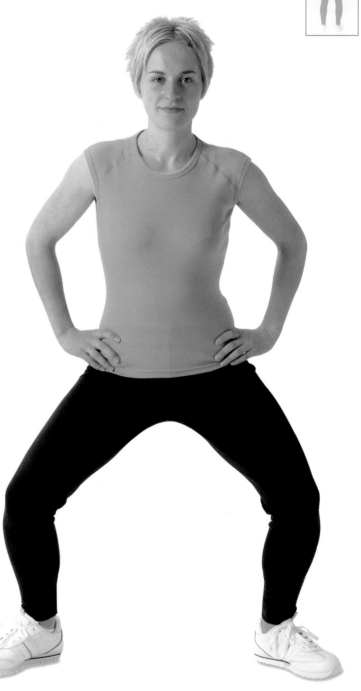

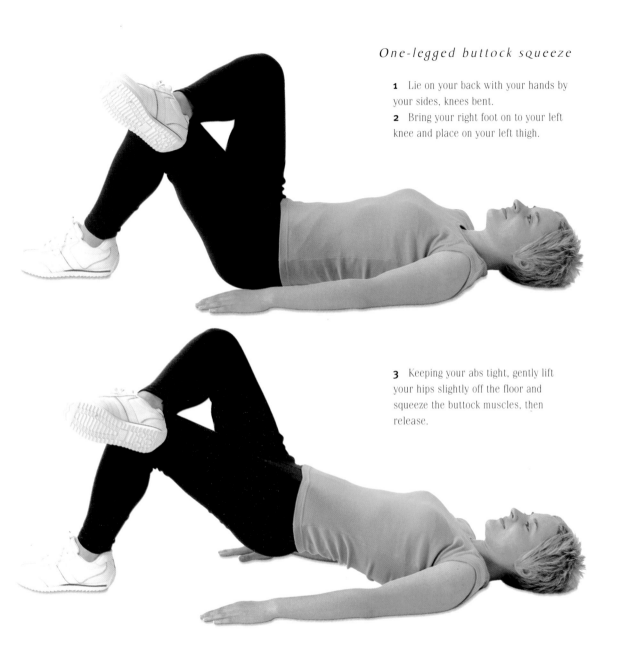

One-legged buttock squeeze

1 Lie on your back with your hands by your sides, knees bent.

2 Bring your right foot on to your left knee and place on your left thigh.

3 Keeping your abs tight, gently lift your hips slightly off the floor and squeeze the buttock muscles, then release.

4 Do one set (8–12 repetitions), then repeat on the other leg.

Remember …
- *Don't over-arch your back.*
- *Keep your hips still.*
- *Abs are held in tight.*

Straight-legged outer thigh raise

1 Lie on your side with your underneath leg bent and the top leg straight, hips facing forward and your body in a straight line.

2 Rest your head in one hand and place the other hand on the floor in front of you for support.

3 Gently raise the top leg (not too high), then lower.

4 Do one set (8–12 repetitions), then repeat on the other side.

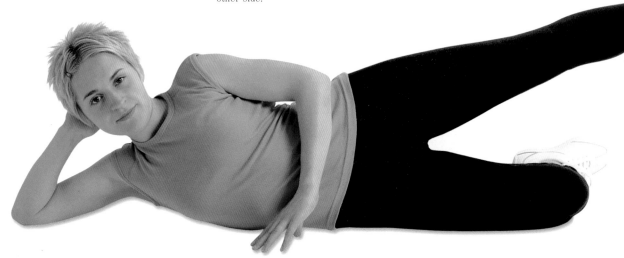

Remember …
- *Hips, knees and toes face forward.*
- *Keep the knee of the extended leg slightly bent.*
- *Squeeze your buttocks.*
- *Abs are held in tight.*

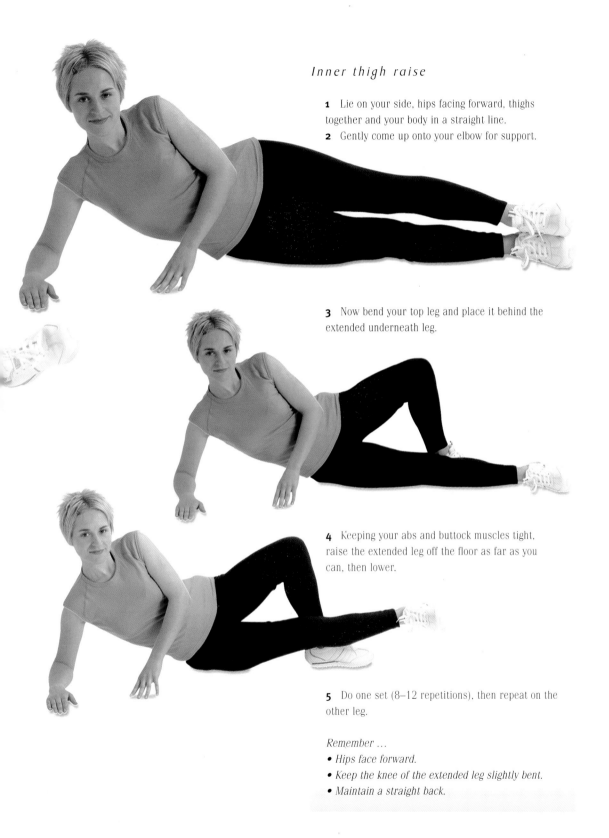

Inner thigh raise

1 Lie on your side, hips facing forward, thighs together and your body in a straight line.

2 Gently come up onto your elbow for support.

3 Now bend your top leg and place it behind the extended underneath leg.

4 Keeping your abs and buttock muscles tight, raise the extended leg off the floor as far as you can, then lower.

5 Do one set (8–12 repetitions), then repeat on the other leg.

Remember ...
- *Hips face forward.*
- *Keep the knee of the extended leg slightly bent.*
- *Maintain a straight back.*

bum
stretches...*intermediate*

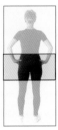

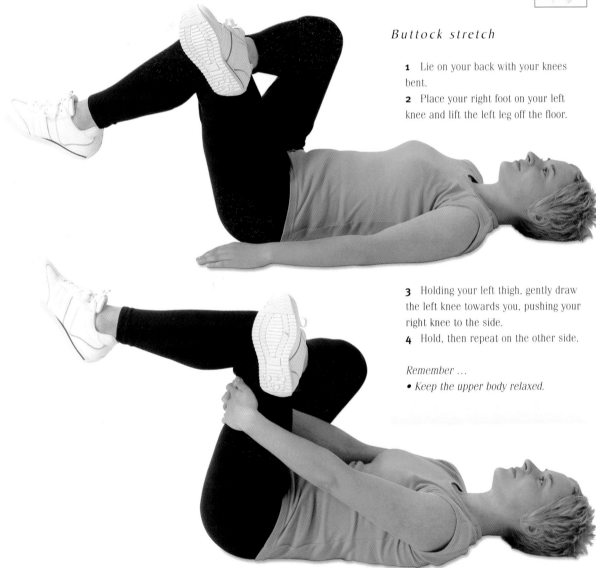

Buttock stretch

1 Lie on your back with your knees bent.

2 Place your right foot on your left knee and lift the left leg off the floor.

3 Holding your left thigh, gently draw the left knee towards you, pushing your right knee to the side.

4 Hold, then repeat on the other side.

Remember ...
• *Keep the upper body relaxed.*

Quad/front of thigh stretch

1 Lie on your side with your legs together and extended, keeping your knees slightly bent.

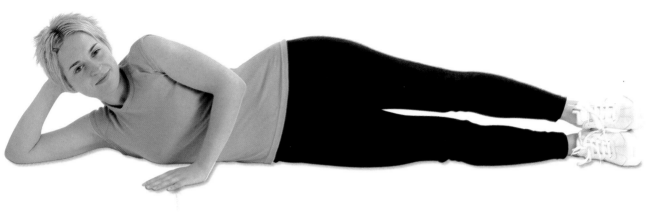

2 Bend your top leg back and bring your top hand to meet your heel.
3 Gently bring your heel closer to your bottom, tilting your pelvis slightly forward as you do so.

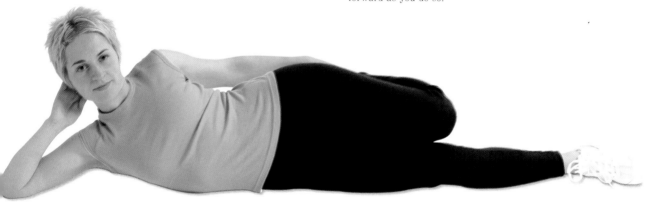

4 Hold, then repeat on the other side.

Remember …
- *Thighs remain parallel.*
- *Don't pull too hard on your knee.*
- *Your body is in a straight line.*

HOLD THESE STRETCHES FOR **6–10** SECONDS IN THE WARM-UP, GRADUALLY BUILDING UP TO **30** SECONDS IN THE COOL-DOWN

Outer thigh/back stretch

1 Sit on the floor with both your legs extended to the front.

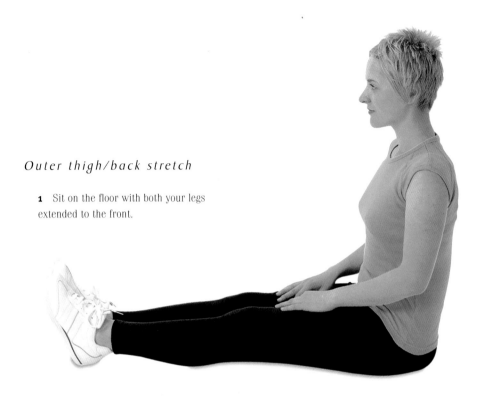

2 Bend your left leg and cross it over your right leg.

3 Keeping your back straight, bring your right arm over to the outside of your left knee, turning your upper body to the left, and gently press your left knee in towards your body.

4 Hold, then repeat on the other side.

Remember ...
• *Your hips and buttocks stay on the floor.*

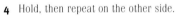

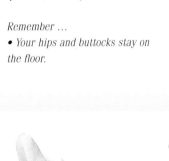

Hamstring stretch

1 Sit on the floor with both legs extended to the front.

2 Bend one leg in so that the knee falls to the side and the foot faces the inner thigh of the straight leg.

3 Keeping your body in line with that leg, gently ease forward, and place your hands on the floor on either side of the leg.

4 Hold, then repeat on the other side. You should feel a stretch in the back of the thigh.

Remember …
- *Lean forward from your hips.*
- *Your back is flat.*
- *Don't bounce.*
- *Abs are held in tight.*

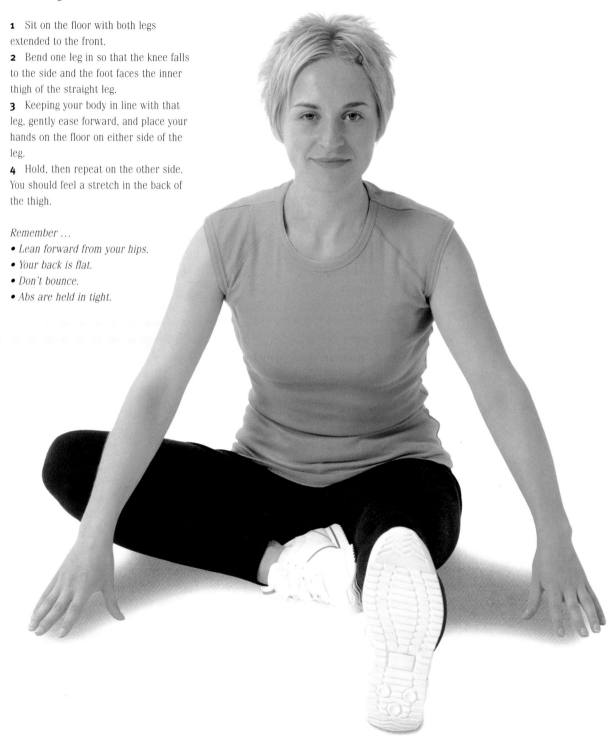

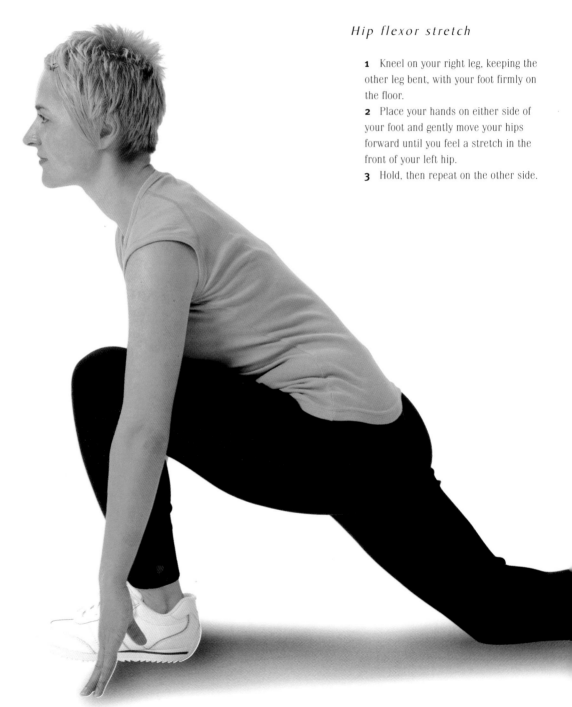

Hip flexor stretch

1 Kneel on your right leg, keeping the other leg bent, with your foot firmly on the floor.

2 Place your hands on either side of your foot and gently move your hips forward until you feel a stretch in the front of your left hip.

3 Hold, then repeat on the other side.

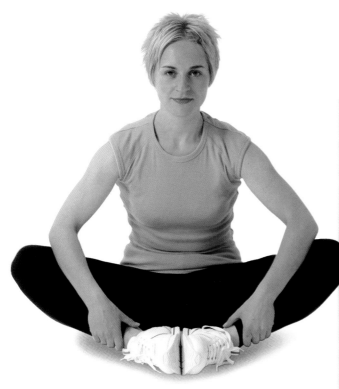

Inner thigh stretch

1 Sit with the soles of your feet together and let your knees drop down to the side.

2 Hold on loosely to your calves or feet and let your elbows gently push down on the fleshy part of your knees.

Remember ...
* *Keep your back straight, chest lifted.*
* *Press your knees only as far as is comfortable.*

NOTE: To increase the stretch, bring your feet closer to the groin.

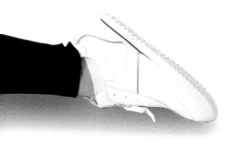

bum programme

Spend about 30 seconds on each exercise on each side (when worked separately).

Warm-up

1 Pelvic tilt
2 Hip circles
3 Knee bends
4 Toe taps, side and behind
5 Marching on the spot until you feel warm
6 Stretch
Hold each stretch for 6–10 seconds:
* Hamstring stretch
* Quad stretch

Toning exercises

1 Wide squat
2 One-legged buttock squeeze
3 Straight-legged outer thigh raise
4 Inner thigh raise
5 Stretch
Hold each stretch for 15–30 seconds:
* Buttock stretch
* Quad stretch
* Outer thigh/back stretch
* Hamstring stretch
* Hip flexor stretch
* Inner thigh stretch

tum
exercises...*intermediate*

 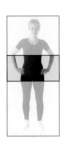

10 MINS

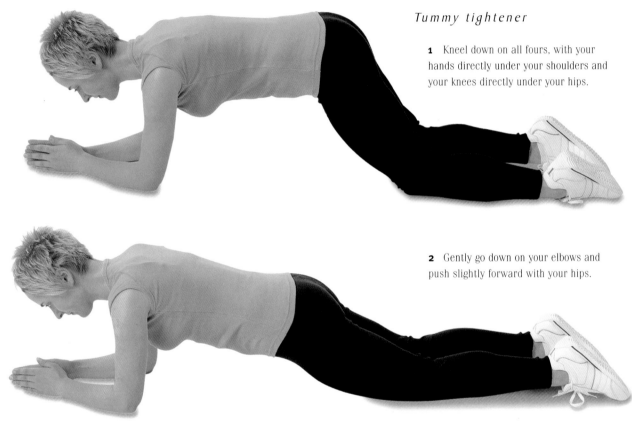

Tummy tightener

1 Kneel down on all fours, with your hands directly under your shoulders and your knees directly under your hips.

2 Gently go down on your elbows and push slightly forward with your hips.

3 Hold your abs in tight.
4 Hold for 30 seconds, building up to 1 minute.

Remember …
* *Breathe.*
* *Keep your back flat and your bottom down.*
* *Your elbows are directly under your shoulders.*

Curl-up

1 Lie on the floor with your feet hip-width apart and firmly on the floor, your knees bent.

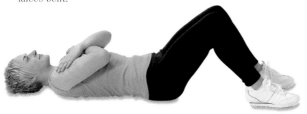

2 Cross your hands over your chest. Tilt your pelvis to a neutral position and tighten your abs. Using your tummy muscles, gently lift your shoulders off the floor, then lower.

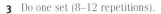

3 Do one set (8–12 repetitions).

Remember …
* *Breathe out when you come up, breathe in when you lower.*
* *Relax your head and neck and keep your chin off your chest.*
* *The movement should be fluid and continuous.*
* *Your back remains on the floor at all times.*

Waist tightener/oblique curl

1 Lie on the floor with your feet hip-width apart and firmly on the floor, your knees bent.
2 Bring your right ankle across your left knee.
3 Place your left hand behind your head, with your elbow bent.
4 Place the other hand on the floor for support.
5 Tighten your abs and slowly curl up and over, bringing your left arm to meet your right knee, then lower.
6 Do one set (8–12 repetitions), then repeat on the other side.

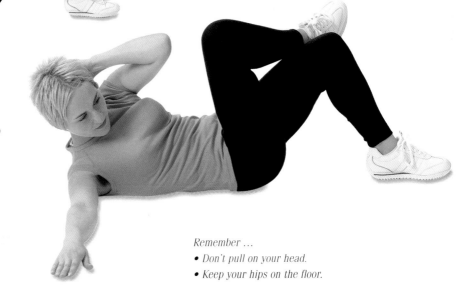

Remember …
* *Don't pull on your head.*
* *Keep your hips on the floor.*

tum

stretches...*intermediate*

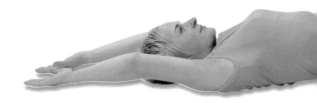

Reverse curl

1 Lie on the floor with your legs raised, knees slightly bent and your ankles crossed over one another so that your knees are directly over your tummy.

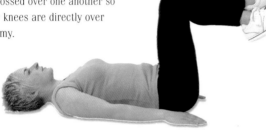

2 Your arms are by your sides, palms down.

3 Tighten your abs.

4 Gently tilt your pelvis up towards the ceiling by bringing your knees towards your chest, then lower (it's a small, rolling action rather than a pushing-up action).

5 Do one set (8–10 repetitions).

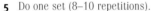
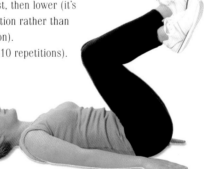

Remember ...
- *Breathe out when you come up, breathe in when you lower.*
- *Don't swing your legs.*
- *Keep your head and neck relaxed.*
- *Squeeze your abs tight.*

Full body stretch

1 Lie on your back with your arms extended above your head.

2 Gently stretch and lengthen your body, right through your fingertips and down to your toes.

3 Hold for a minimum of 10 seconds, gradually building up to 30, then gently release and slowly bring your arms down by your side.

Remember ...
- *Breathe gently.*
- *Don't over-arch your back.*

Note: Your lower back may come gently off the floor.

Note: It's a good idea to train a different part of the tummy on alternate days to get the maximum benefit. For example, Monday, upper abs (curl-up), Tuesday, obliques (elbow to knee), Wednesday, lower abs (reverse curl). This will also prevent you from getting bored with the programme – and giving up.

Waist stretch

1 Sit with your legs straight out in front of you.

2 Bend your right leg and cross it over your left leg.

3 Bring your left elbow over to the outside of your right knee, keeping the right hand on the ground for support.

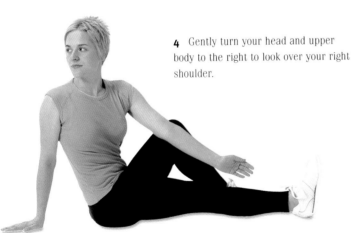

4 Gently turn your head and upper body to the right to look over your right shoulder.

5 Hold for 15 seconds.

6 Repeat on the other side.

Remember …
• *Keep your hips and bottom on the floor.*

tum programme

Spend about 30 seconds on each exercise.

Warm-up

1 Pelvic tilt
2 Waist twists
3 Spinal curl
4 Side bends
5 Marching on the spot until you feel warm
6 Stretch
Hold for 6–10 seconds:
• Full body stretch

Toning exercises

1 Tummy tightener
2 Curl-up
3 Waist tightener/oblique curl
4 Reverse curl
5 Stretch
Hold each stretch for 15–30 seconds:
• Full body stretch
• Waist stretch

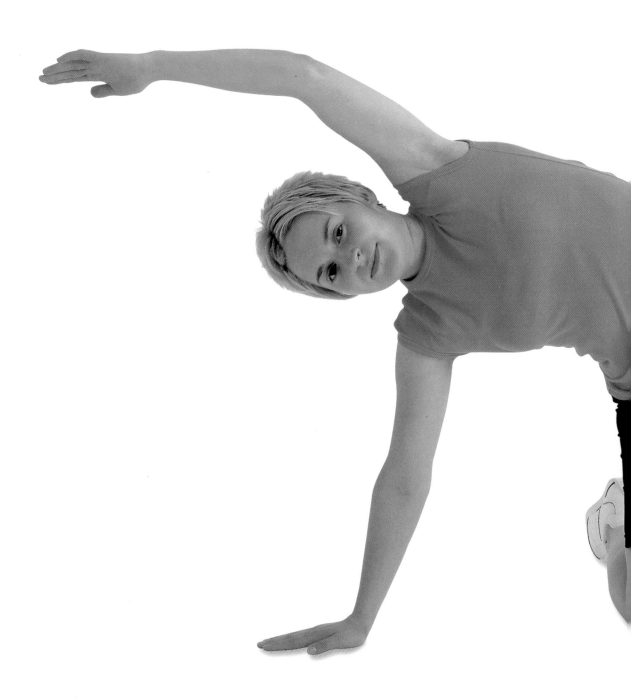

10 AdvancedWorkout

Now that you are ready to tackle the advanced workout, you should know how to perform both the bum and the tum exercises correctly, using all the right muscles. The results of your efforts will really be starting to show, so you should be feeling much more confident and highly motivated to continue. As you embark on the advanced routine, make every repetition count as you give your buttock muscles a challenging workout. The exercises in this section are more difficult than those in the earlier sections, and now that your bum and tum muscles have become so much stronger, it is even more important to remember to keep the movements slow and controlled. And remember to breathe, too – it's easy to forget about your breathing as you concentrate on working harder, and then wonder why you suddenly collapse in a breathless heap!

bum

exercises...*advanced*

 10 MINS

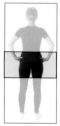

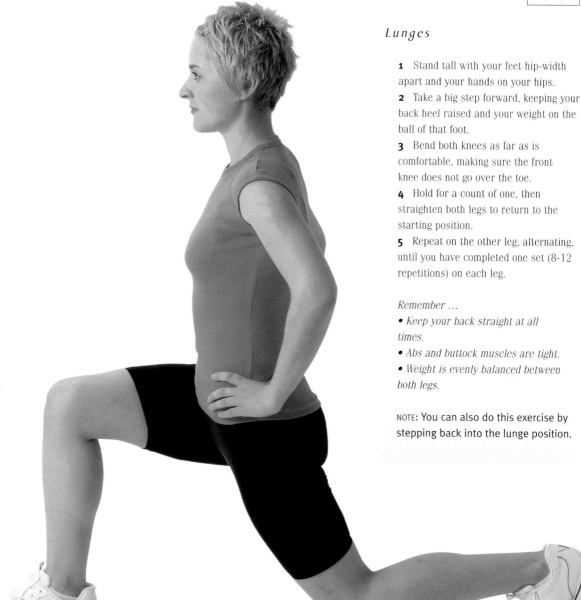

Lunges

1 Stand tall with your feet hip-width apart and your hands on your hips.

2 Take a big step forward, keeping your back heel raised and your weight on the ball of that foot.

3 Bend both knees as far as is comfortable, making sure the front knee does not go over the toe.

4 Hold for a count of one, then straighten both legs to return to the starting position.

5 Repeat on the other leg, alternating, until you have completed one set (8-12 repetitions) on each leg.

Remember ...
* *Keep your back straight at all times.*
* *Abs and buttock muscles are tight.*
* *Weight is evenly balanced between both legs.*

NOTE: You can also do this exercise by stepping back into the lunge position.

Squats and side leg raises

1 Stand with your feet hip-width apart, toes facing forward.

2 Place your hands on your hips.

3 Bend your knees like you're about to sit down in a chair, sticking your bottom out to the back.

4 Push through the heels to come up and as you do so raise your right leg to the side (not too high).

5 Hold and squeeze your buttocks and outer thigh muscles.

6 Squat down, then repeat on the other side.

7 Do one set (8–12 repetitions) on each leg.

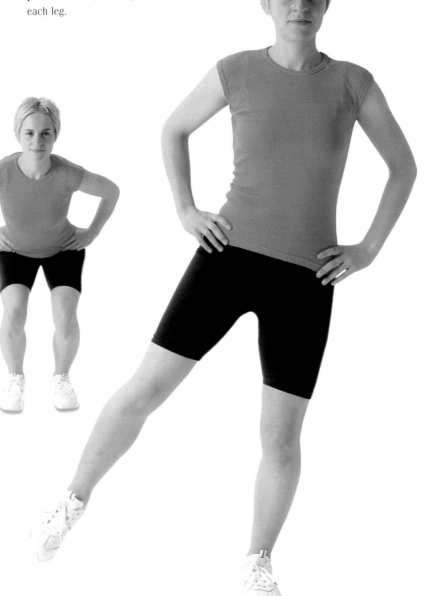

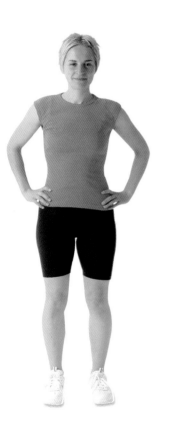

Remember …
* *Your posture – chest is high, abs are tight.*
* *Toes and knees face forward.*
* *Don't lock your knees.*

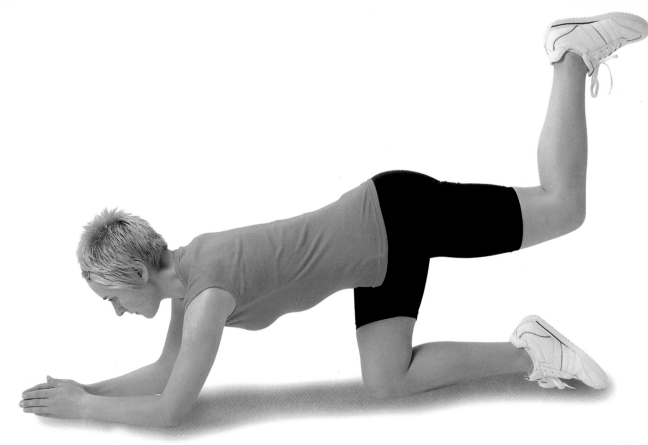

Kneeling buttock tightener

1 Kneel on all fours in a box position with your hands on the floor.

2 Gently go down on to your elbows, extend one leg to the back and bend at the knee so that it's in line with your hips and the heel is facing the ceiling. Your back is flat (this is the starting position).

3 Squeezing your buttock muscles, gently raise your leg, then lower to the starting position.

4 Do one set (8–12 repetitions), then repeat on the other leg.

Remember ...
- *Don't move your hips.*
- *Keep your heel facing the ceiling.*
- *Make sure your back is flat.*

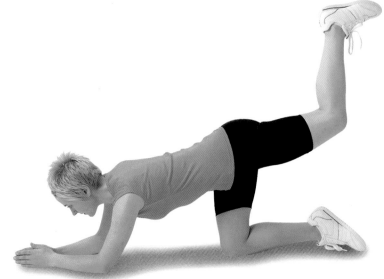

Inner thigh raise

1 Lie on your side, hips facing forward, thighs together and your body in a straight line.

2 Gently come up on to your elbow for support.

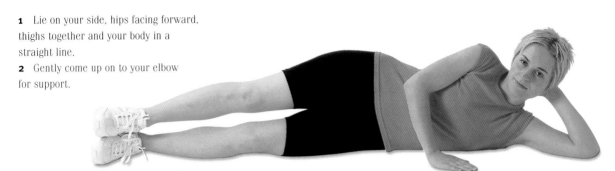

3 Now bend your top leg and place your foot on the inner part of the bottom leg.

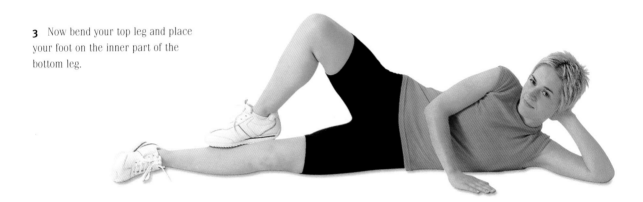

4 Raise the lower leg off the floor, then lower.

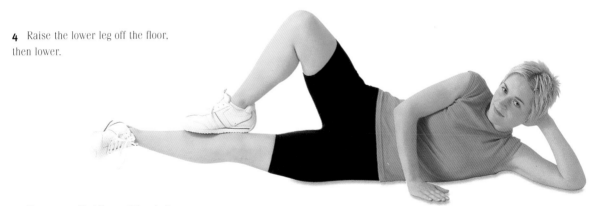

5 Do one set (8–12 repetitions), then repeat on the other leg.

Remember …
* *Hips face forward.*
* *Body remains aligned.*

bum
stretches...*advanced*

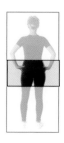

Quad/front of thigh stretch

1 Lie on your stomach and rest your head on your right arm.

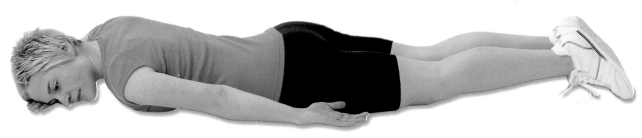

2 Bend your left leg and reach for your left foot with your left hand.
3 Gently pull towards your buttocks until you feel a stretch in the front of your thigh.

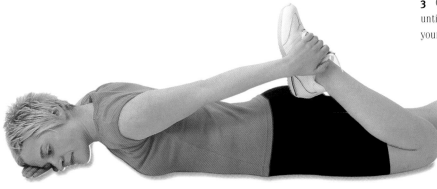

4 Hold, then repeat on the other side.

Remember ...
• *Keep your hips pressed into the floor.*

> ! HOLD THESE STRETCHES FOR **6–10** SECONDS IN THE WARM-UP, GRADUALLY BUILDING UP TO **30** SECONDS IN THE COOL-DOWN

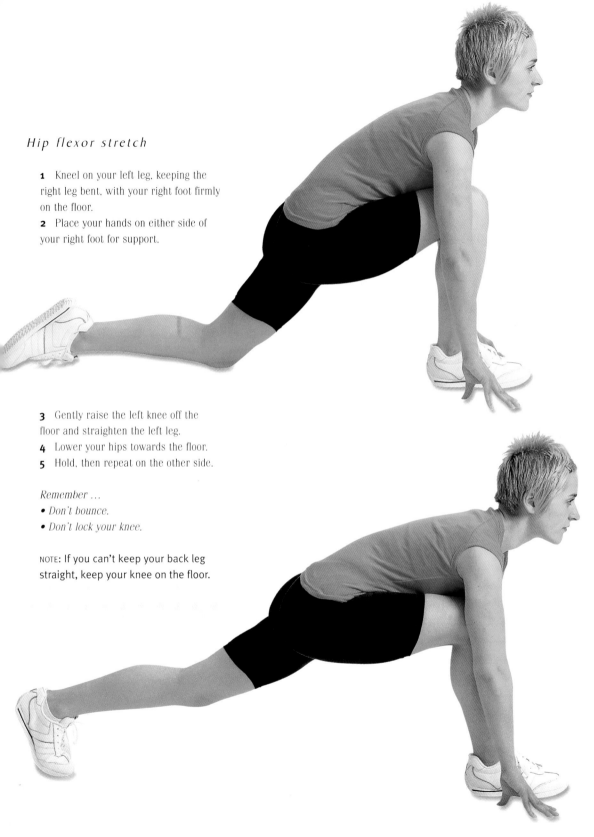

Hip flexor stretch

1 Kneel on your left leg, keeping the right leg bent, with your right foot firmly on the floor.

2 Place your hands on either side of your right foot for support.

3 Gently raise the left knee off the floor and straighten the left leg.

4 Lower your hips towards the floor.

5 Hold, then repeat on the other side.

Remember …
- *Don't bounce.*
- *Don't lock your knee.*

NOTE: If you can't keep your back leg straight, keep your knee on the floor.

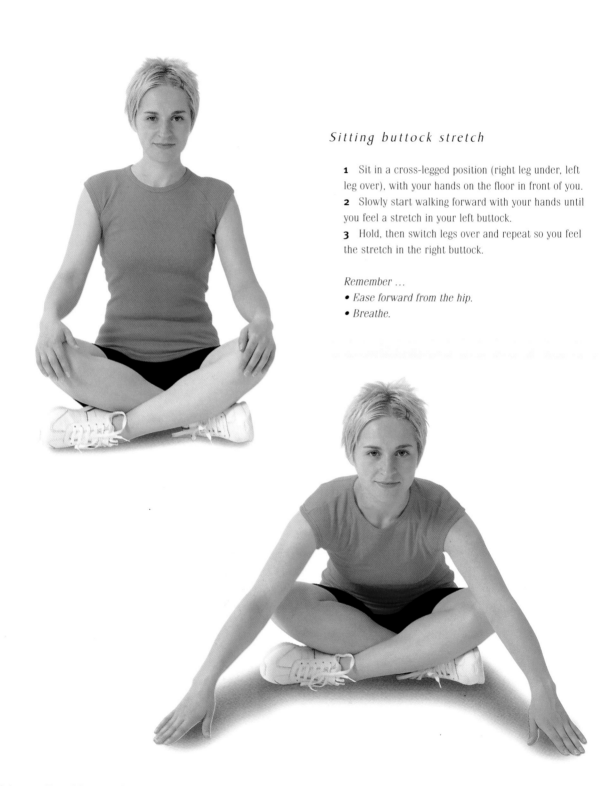

Sitting buttock stretch

1 Sit in a cross-legged position (right leg under, left leg over), with your hands on the floor in front of you.
2 Slowly start walking forward with your hands until you feel a stretch in your left buttock.
3 Hold, then switch legs over and repeat so you feel the stretch in the right buttock.

Remember …
• *Ease forward from the hip.*
• *Breathe.*

Straddle stretch

1 Sit on the floor with your legs wide apart, your hands on the floor in front of you.
2 Slowly start walking your hands forward, bending forward from the hips until you feel a stretch on the inside and back of your thighs.
3 Hold.

Remember …
* *Don't bounce.*
* *Only go as far as is comfortable.*

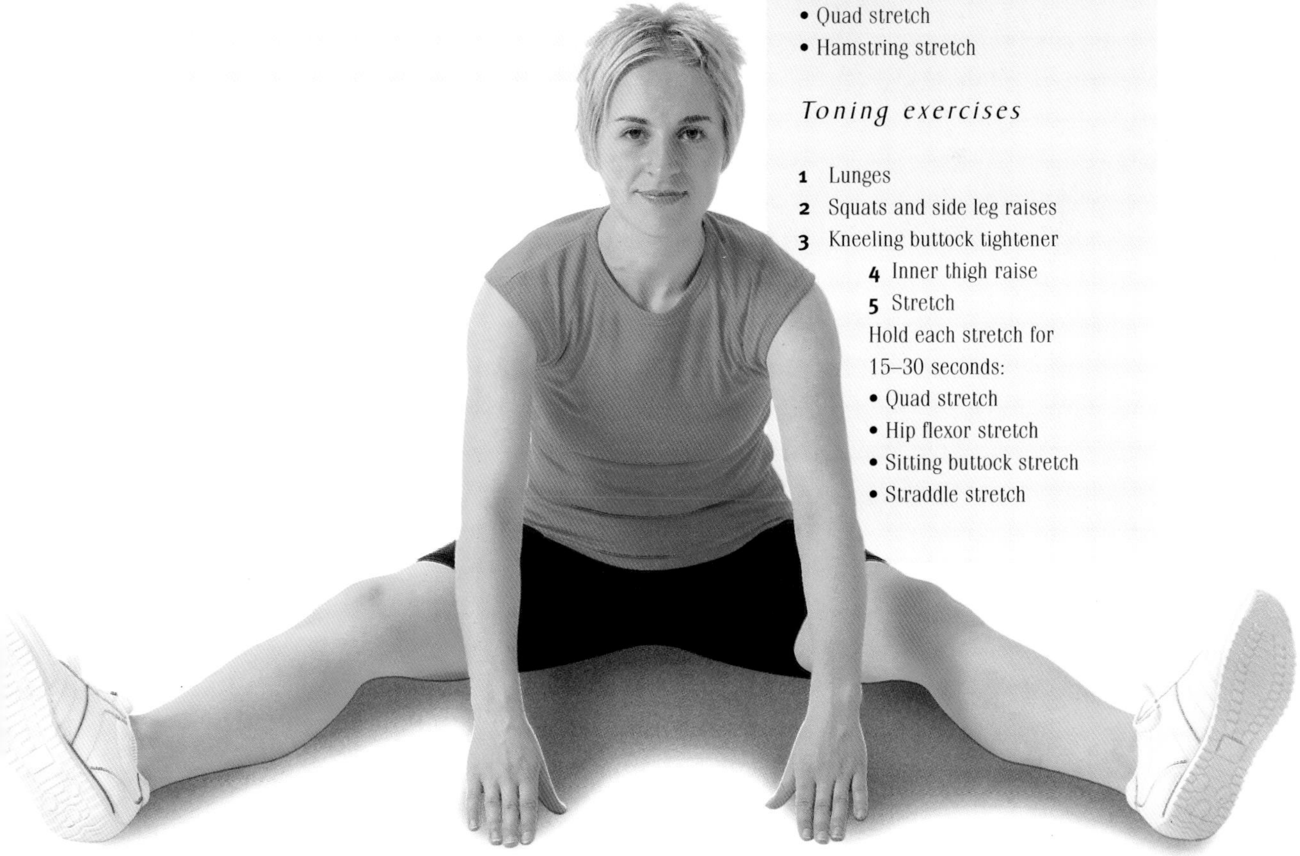

bum programme

Spend about 30 seconds on each exercise on each side (when worked separately).

Warm-up

1 Pelvic tilt
2 Hip circles
3 Knee bends
4 Toe taps, side and behind
5 Marching on the spot until you feel warm
6 Stretch
Hold each stretch for 6–10 seconds:
* Quad stretch
* Hamstring stretch

Toning exercises

1 Lunges
2 Squats and side leg raises
3 Kneeling buttock tightener
4 Inner thigh raise
5 Stretch
Hold each stretch for 15–30 seconds:
* Quad stretch
* Hip flexor stretch
* Sitting buttock stretch
* Straddle stretch

tum

exercises...*advanced*

 10 MINS

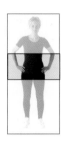

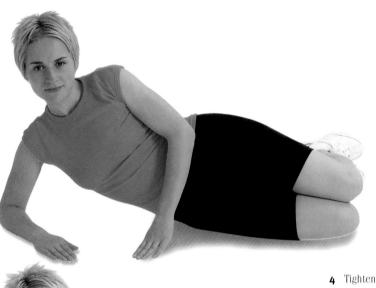

Waist tightener

1 Lie on your side with your body in a straight line.
2 Bend your knees slightly.
3 Place your elbow underneath your shoulder and your other hand in front of you on the floor.

4 Tighten your abs and ease your hips off the ground.
5 Take your hand off the floor and place it on your side.
6 Hold for 15 seconds, building up to 30 seconds.

Remember …
• *Keep your body in a straight line, knees slightly bent.*
• *Leave your hand on the floor if you have trouble balancing in this position.*

NOTE: If you have shoulder problems, check with your doctor before trying this exercise.

Full-length tummy tightener/the plank

1 Kneel on all fours, then go down on to your elbows.
2 Gently straighten your right leg to the back, your toes curled under, then straighten your left leg in the same way, so that both feet are together.
3 Pull your abs in tight and lower your hips.
4 Hold for 15 to 30 seconds, building up to 1 minute.

Remember …
• *Breathe.*
• *Keep your head in line with your body and your back flat.*

NOTE: If you feel any strain in your back, either widen your stance or lower your knees to the floor as demonstrated in the Intermediate Workout.

Advanced curl-up

1 Lie on the floor with your feet hip-width apart and firmly on the floor, your knees bent.
2 Tilt your pelvis to a neutral position and tighten your abs.

Remember …
• *Breathe out when you come up, breathe in when you lower.*
• *Relax your head and neck and keep your chin off your chest.*
• *The movement should be fluid and continuous.*
• *Your back remains on the floor at all times.*

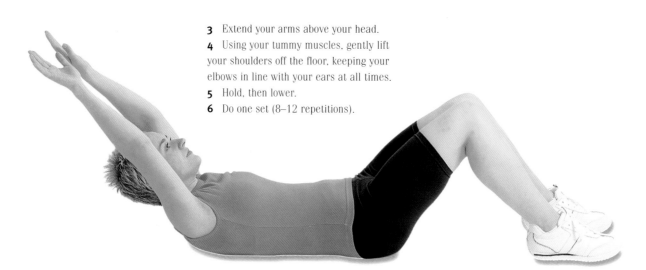

3 Extend your arms above your head.
4 Using your tummy muscles, gently lift your shoulders off the floor, keeping your elbows in line with your ears at all times.
5 Hold, then lower.
6 Do one set (8–12 repetitions).

Reverse curl

1 Lie on the floor with your arms by your sides, palms down, and your legs straight up in the air.

2 Keep your knees slightly bent and your feet crossed at the ankles.

3 Tighten your abs and gently tilt your pelvis up so your bottom comes off the floor, then lower.

4 Do one set (8–10 repetitions).

Remember …
* *Breathe.*
* *Keep your legs still – try not to sway back and forth.*
* *The movement is small and controlled.*

NOTE: You can have your arms extended above your head, if you like.

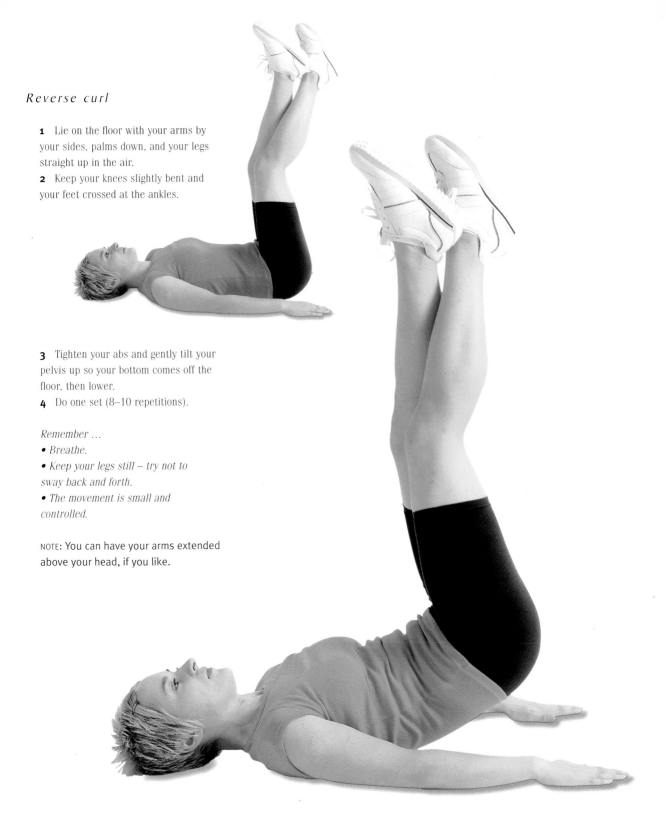

tum
stretches...*advanced*

Abdominal stretch

1 Lie on your stomach, place your hands on the floor in front with your arms extended in front, your elbows slightly bent.

2 Gently push on your hands and lift your

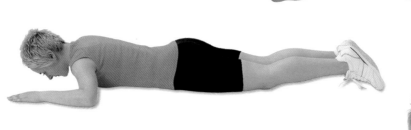

shoulders and head off the floor until you feel a stretch in your abdominal muscles.

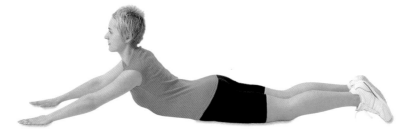

3 Hold for a minimum of 10 seconds.

Remember ...
* *Look straight ahead when you lift your head.*
* *Keep your hips and feet on the floor.*
* *Don't strain your back – only come up as far as is comfortable.*

Side stretch

1 Kneel on your right knee, straighten your left leg to the side.
2 Place your right hand on the floor on the right side and gently bring your left arm over your head to stretch the side of the body.
3 Hold for a minimum of 10 seconds. Repeat on the other side.

Remember …
• *Your right knee is directly under your right hip.*

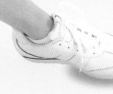

tum programme

Spend about 30 seconds on each exercise on each side (when worked separately).

Warm-up

1 Pelvic tilt
2 Waist twists
3 Side bends
4 Spinal curl
5 Marching on the spot until you feel warm
6 Stretch
Hold the stretch for 15–30 seconds
• Full body stretch

Toning exercises

1 Waist tightener
2 Full-length tummy tightener/ the plank
3 Curl-up
4 Reverse curl
5 Stretch:
Hold each stretch for 15–30 seconds:
• Ab stretch
  • Side stretch

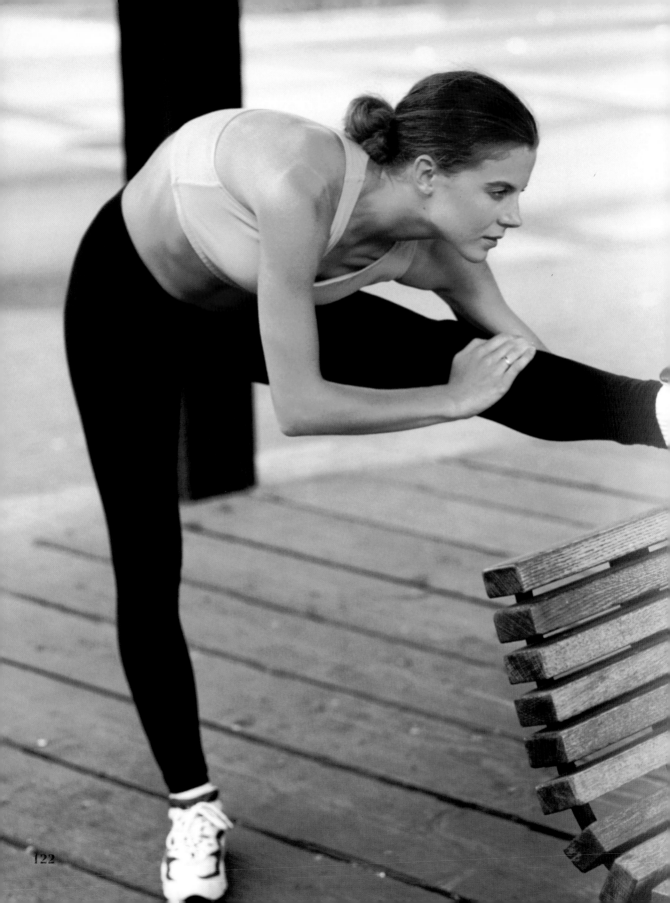

11 TheWayAhead

So that's it! Congratulations! You've completed the ten-minute tone-up programme and are now enjoying the results – improved posture and a toned (and stunning!) bum and tum, as well as a new poise and confidence. You will probably also notice that you have become much stronger, with more stamina and fewer aches and pains. Daily activities seem easier, particularly lifting, climbing stairs and bending, and you will be more flexible as a result of stretching at the end of every session. In addition to all this is the satisfaction you will feel from sticking to a plan, and a fantastic sense of well-being because exercise releases the body's 'feel-good' hormones, endorphins. You've worked very hard to achieve this new you, so what should you do now to stay fit?

The answer is simple – keep it up!

2 ten-minute *toning* programme

To keep up the good work and get the best from toning your bum and tum, exercise each muscle group two to three times a week. Divide your week into two toning sessions and one posture session.

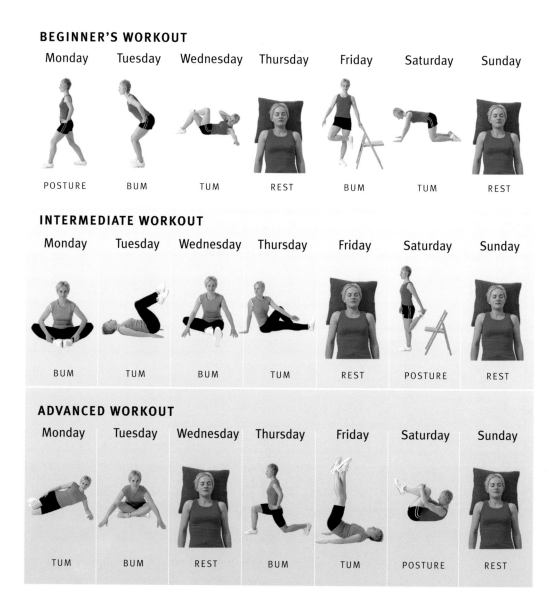

BEGINNER'S WORKOUT

Monday	Tuesday	Wednesday	Thursday	Friday	Saturday	Sunday
POSTURE	BUM	TUM	REST	BUM	TUM	REST

INTERMEDIATE WORKOUT

Monday	Tuesday	Wednesday	Thursday	Friday	Saturday	Sunday
BUM	TUM	BUM	TUM	REST	POSTURE	REST

ADVANCED WORKOUT

Monday	Tuesday	Wednesday	Thursday	Friday	Saturday	Sunday
TUM	BUM	REST	BUM	TUM	POSTURE	REST

keeping your *new shape*

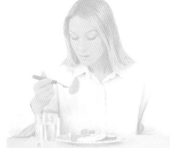

Once you've achieved the bum and tum you want, you'll need to maintain it. If you like, you can work out less – perhaps two or three sessions a week on each muscle group. You can achieve this by following the exercise plan on page 126, but make sure you continue to work hard and keep up the intensity. Or you can take on a few of the challenges below. And most of all, enjoy the new you!

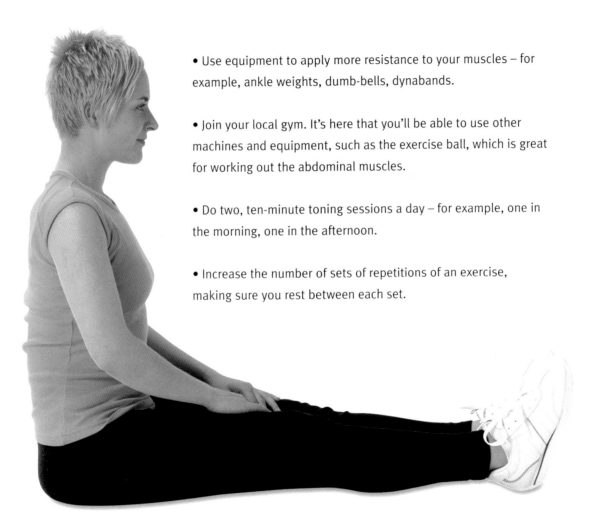

• Use equipment to apply more resistance to your muscles – for example, ankle weights, dumb-bells, dynabands.

• Join your local gym. It's here that you'll be able to use other machines and equipment, such as the exercise ball, which is great for working out the abdominal muscles.

• Do two, ten-minute toning sessions a day – for example, one in the morning, one in the afternoon.

• Increase the number of sets of repetitions of an exercise, making sure you rest between each set.

exercise *plan*

Here's a simple weekly routine you can follow. Work up to two or three sets of 8–12 repetitions.

Morning

Evening

MONDAY

- Outer thigh raise
- Inner thigh raise
- Stretch

- Abs
- Stretch

TUESDAY

- One-legged buttock squeeze
- Squats
- Stretch

WEDNESDAY

- Abs
- Stretch

THURSDAY

- Kneeling buttock tightener
- Lunges
- Stretch

FRIDAY

- Outer thigh raise
- Inner thigh raise
- Stretch

- Abs
- Stretch

SATURDAY/SUNDAY

- Rest

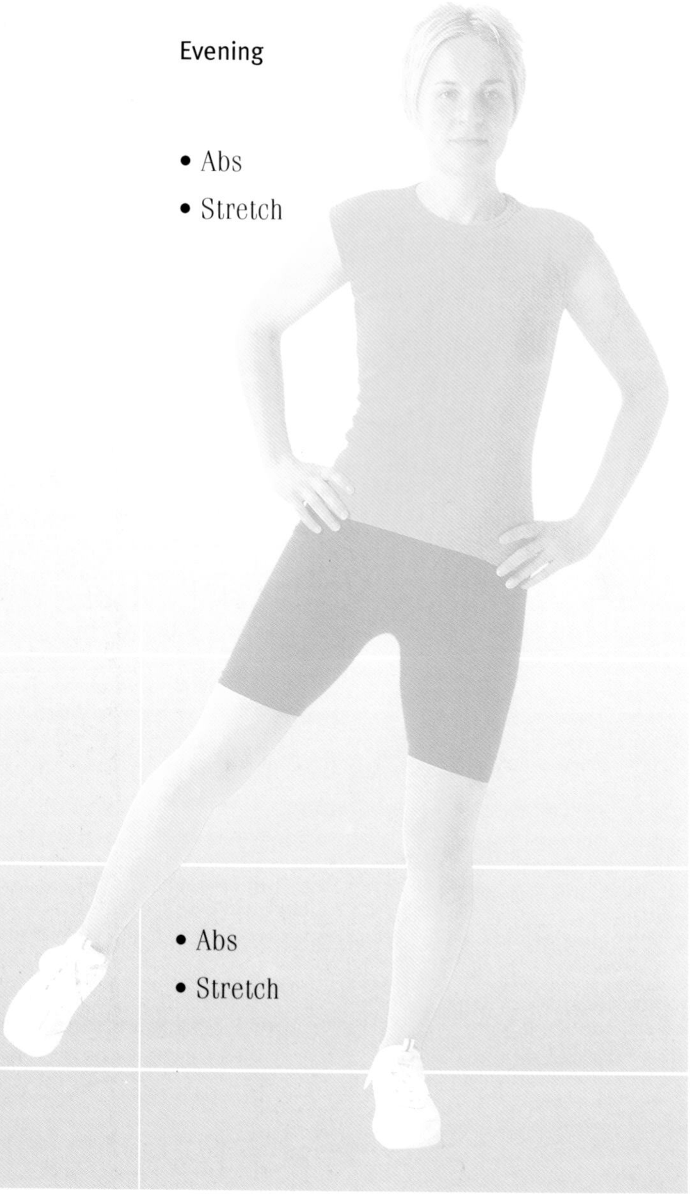

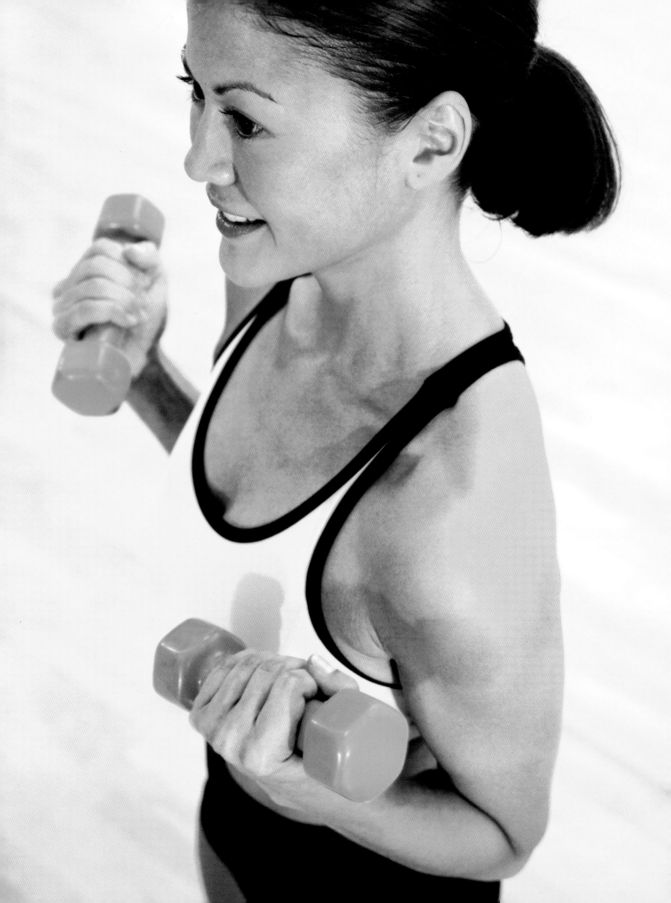

index